A STATE OF EMERGENCY

D0865996

A STATE OF EMERGENCY

The Story of Ireland's Covid Crisis

Richard Chambers

HarperCollins*Ireland*

HarperCollins*Ireland*
1st Floor, Watermarque Building, Ringsend Road
Dublin 4, Ireland

a division of
HarperCollins*Publishers*
1 London Bridge Street
London SE1 9GF
UK

www.harpercollins.co.uk

First published by HarperCollins*Ireland* 2021

1 3 5 7 9 10 8 6 4 2

© Richard Chambers 2021

Richard Chambers asserts the moral right to
be identified as the author of this work

Photographs courtesy of the author unless otherwise stated

A catalogue record of this book is available from the British Library

ISBN 978-0-00-850282-9

Typeset in Minion by Palimpsest Book Production Ltd, Falkirk, Stirlingshire
Printed and Bound in the UK using 100% Renewable Electricity
at CPI Group (UK) Ltd

All rights reserved. No part of this publication may be
reproduced, stored in a retrieval system, or transmitted,
in any form or by any means, electronic, mechanical,
photocopying, recording or otherwise, without the prior
permission of the publishers.

MIX
Paper from
responsible sources
FSC™ C007454

This book is produced from independently certified FSC™ paper to ensure
responsible forest management.

For more information visit: www.harpercollins.co.uk/green

Dedicated to the healthcare workers who saved countless lives and in memory of those no longer with us.

Contents

PART I

Chapter 1: The Beginning

Dillinger's Restaurant, Ranelagh, 10 January 2020

Tony Holohan, his wife and two teenage children were in Dillinger's in Ranelagh for dinner. Surrounded by the buzz of laughter and groups of young diners meeting over cocktails and craft beers, Holohan was preoccupied. He couldn't fully concentrate on the meal, digging at it with his fork, his mind wandering to what was happening in China. He'd read a medical journal article on clusters of pneumonia of unknown origin in Wuhan and he did not like what he was hearing. 'If something is going to knock us over, this is it.'

By early January, Holohan, Ireland's Chief Medical Officer (CMO), had casually contacted a number of his closest colleagues, a sounding board of experts working across the health sector who would tell him straight if they were worried about this siren blaring in the East. He'd call Cillian De Gascun, Director of the National Virus Reference Laboratory (NVRL) at University College Dublin (UCD); Ronan Glynn, Deputy CMO; Kevin Kelleher, Assistant National Director for Public Health at the Health Service Executive (HSE); and John Cuddihy, the interim leader of the Health Protection Surveillance Centre (HPSC).

They'd have the odd chat in the evenings, talking about this new virus, what stood out to each of them, the links to a seafood

3

Leabharlanna Poiblí Chathair Baile Átha Cliath
Dublin City Public Libraries

market, the lack of transparency from China, the worrying signs of severe illness, the question mark around human-to-human transmission, and the fact that there was nobody in the world with any immunity to this thing.

The weekend of 25–26 January, Holohan was down in Limerick for his sister's fiftieth birthday. On the way back to Dublin, with his daughter driving the car, he called his insiders once more. It had just dawned on him that firmer action was now needed.

'Guys, I think we need to have a NPHET meeting. We need to formally organize.'

NPHET, the National Public Health Emergency Team, was not a new construct. There had been a number of NPHETs before. There had been NPHETs for moments of concern including the H1N1 swine flu, and just the previous year, 2019, for the CPE superbug scare. This time was shaping up to be very different.

The meeting was held in the Department of Health's upstairs boardroom on 27 January. Eleven people attended, led by Holohan. As the officials came together, there was a touch of excitement in the air. 'It's always nice to be in the room,' says Cillian De Gascun, who looked around the conference room high above central Dublin, as small talk filled the air. Officials chatted to each other before the meeting and on their way out. Some were familiar to each other, others were close colleagues who'd served years together in health services. 'Agh, it could go the way of SARS or MERS,' some officials reassured themselves; 'there was a feeling that even though we had convened, this could be a short-lived thing'.

The gathering was short, a check-in more than a crisis engagement. An opportunity to get faces in the room together. Boxes were ticked. The HSE's Emergency Management office said it would have a sufficient supply of personal protective equipment (PPE) for the 'coming weeks', with contracts in place to access more should it be required.

It was a meeting few people took notice of. There was no media reporting of the convening of NPHET or the HSE's National Crisis Management Team for a number of days. All attention was on a hotly contested general election campaign. Politicians had yet to see the storm clouds gather.

* * * *

'This one could get out of the bag.'

Professor Máire Connolly had been around long enough to know that something different was happening here. The Galway woman is one of the foremost experts in emerging infectious diseases and pandemic preparedness in Ireland, or anywhere for that matter. She had worked for many years in a lead role with the World Health Organization (WHO) and few people have stacked up as many airmiles in tracking global disease threats and natural disasters – she's been in Afghanistan, Kosovo, Iraq, Gaza, Uganda, Iran, Indonesia, to name just a few. In 2005, a *New York Times* profile interview focused on the emergency relief work that took her, and often her husband, Dr Mike Ryan, also of the WHO, across the globe, often in separate directions. It was dangerous work. Connolly was confronted by soldiers brandishing guns in East Timor who didn't understand her mission to hang mosquito traps. 'Can't you two ever stay in one place at the same time?' her mother asked her in those days.

More than anyone else in the country, having led the PANDEM pandemic response project since leaving the WHO, she understands the risks of communicable diseases. What she heard in January did not sound at all good to her. The Christmas decorations were still up at home as she spoke with her old colleagues in Geneva the day after New Year's Day. The

5

rumblings were not encouraging. One colleague was particularly concerned about data coming from the WHO's office in Beijing. The alarm bells were already sounding for Connolly.

Governments and health departments around the world have tended to look at experts in emerging infectious diseases as shroud wavers. They had sounded the alarm about the swine flu H1N1 and the bird flu H5N1. The sky didn't fall. The world didn't cave when SARS arrived in 2003 or MERS in 2012. Neither did it take notice of the ominous sign that two novel coronaviruses had emerged in a ten-year period. There was little fear of a third.

The hope, and it was a hope, for the global community was that this new virus would go the way of SARS-1 and be controlled, contained, and moved on from within a matter of months.

'The fundamental difference,' says Connolly, was that with SARS, 'if you get infected on day zero and you become sick on day five, you have a week before you become infectious.' With Covid, 'it became clear quite early on in the pandemic that there was transmission going on that wasn't symptomatic – you were transmitting it before you were clinically unwell. If you get infected on day zero, you can end up transmitting the disease on day three and then you become sick on day five. Or you could be someone who doesn't get sick at all and manages to transmit the virus.'

The world had dodged a bullet with SARS-1. With Covid, it would not be so lucky.

This was the root of all that followed. With a new virus, there is a lot to learn, and you have to learn fast. The world's authorities simply didn't get what everyone came to know about the virus in the following months: that it can spread from people who do not have symptoms, or who do not yet have symptoms; that face coverings are an effective measure to control transmission; that it can spread through the air beyond the two-metre close contact boundary.

'It's the risk of fighting the last war,' says Dr Cillian De Gascun, 'and trying to learn from SARS and MERS. This didn't seem to be terribly transmissible at this stage.' It was a lesson that would be hard learned over many weeks and months to come. Only in the spring that followed would public health authorities put into place recommendations on measures like masks and travel. By then it was all very much too late. The virus seeded itself across international travel and gained dominion over Ireland and the wider world.

The Independent Panel for Pandemic Preparedness and Response, commissioned by the WHO to review the early response to this new threat, was damning. This was the twenty-first century's 'Chernobyl moment' and the world's authorities had failed to act swiftly enough to raise the alarm. What followed was a 'lost month', February 2020, when countries began to see cases emerge within their own borders and then, belatedly, put measures in place.

In Ireland, the threshold to be considered a suspect case was high. To be considered a possible case, you would have to display the symptoms of high fever, a cough and shortness of breath and also have travelled from China within the previous fourteen days. The risk of transmission was deemed by the European Centre for Disease Prevention and Control to be 'low'.

* * * *

For Dr Colm Henry, it was the first instance of 'magical thinking', a descriptor that came to define much of the pandemic. Henry, originally from Cavan town, was a geriatrician by speciality in the Mercy University Hospital in Cork and, since April 2018, had been the Chief Clinical Officer of the HSE.

'Magical thinking characterized the whole year for me, meaning that your thinking evolved to what you *wanted* it to

7

be. There was a sense of otherness about it, that it was something that was happening *over there*. The magical thinking began the moment we heard of it, thinking that it belonged someplace else.'

Henry was on holiday in South America when he first noticed the stories about the new virus. His own magical thinking, he says, was along the lines of 'It can't be that bad'; sure wasn't he in a concert hall with hundreds of people and wasn't everything fine?

During his two weeks away, his phone rang with urgent matters from the HSE. 'Strangely enough, none of them were related to Covid-19.' The virus was still very much in the peripheral vision.

* * * *

The first time the Government was alerted to the coronavirus was on 28 January, the day after the first NPHET meeting. Health Minister Simon Harris brought a memo to his colleagues that included advice from the WHO to implement measures to limit the risk of importing cases 'without the unnecessary restriction of international traffic'.

For the ministers around the table, this was all just background noise at this point. One senior minister says, 'The first time the government really became aware from a crystal clear point of view that this was going to be a major deal' would not be for at least another month.

The virus was not a feature of the general election; the airwaves and conversations on doorsteps were dominated by housing and rows over whether or not to commemorate the Royal Irish Constabulary. 'It is quite something, isn't it? If we are really honest, all of us, Ireland wide, we had no sense of this,' says Sinn Féin's leader Mary Lou McDonald. 'I'm assuming that somewhere in officialdom, those in public health and epidemiology had their eyes on the ball, but I can tell you – the political system didn't.'

The civil servants in the Department of Health felt liberated in the political vacuum. They had the space, the bandwidth, to focus on organizing themselves unimpeded against the threat growing in the East.

'I think what would have been different if there hadn't been an election,' says one senior government adviser, 'is that there would have been a structure put in place by Government rather than by officials themselves. Because of the election, the civil servants took over at the very start. Everyone there knew that Harris wasn't going to be the Minister for Health. Leo Varadkar wasn't going to be the Taoiseach. So the civil service were using this as their opportunity to get a bit of power back from the Government and run things the way they saw fit.'

The Department of Health was otherwise, in effect, in sleep mode. 'A lot of things slow down in government departments because ministers aren't in a position to bring forward policy,' says Holohan. 'The only things that happen are the things that simply must happen.'

The Department and its management board was confined to core business. At a meeting in a Miesian Plaza boardroom, in the vacuum of the usual policy-driven objectives, the top civil servants clicked pens and looked at an empty to-do list for the weeks ahead. 'Has anyone got anything at all?' After a brief pause, Holohan chimed in. 'Well, it's funny you should say that,' he said. 'I think I have something.'

* * * *

A dejected Simon Harris was in his office at the Department of Health, stuffing cardboard boxes. He was set for the road. It was the Monday after the election on Friday and the public looked to have called a halt to Fine Gael's nine years in government.

According to people closest to him, he would be checking out. The general election was called to head off a motion of no confidence in him as the Minister for Health, off the back of the hospital overcrowding and trolley crisis. In his own mind, he felt that whatever the outcome of the vote, he would no longer be occupying the minister's office in Miesian Plaza. While the results left an uncertain split between the three largest parties, Harris wanted closure and to move on.

As he packed notes, stationery and personal belongings into boxes to be dropped out to his constituency office, his private secretary stuck her head in the door. 'Are you mad?' she said. 'This could go on for months yet.'

Harris, at thirty-three still a young politician, was facing a crossroads. He'd told his confidantes that he'd do whatever was required to keep things ticking along, but he was on his way out. The office of the Minister for Health is almost right beside the office of the Chief Medical Officer and the offices of many of the senior members of the Department's board of management. Harris's relationship with Tony Holohan appeared to be coming to an abrupt end. It was a relationship that was complicated, to say the least.

The two had worked closely throughout Harris's four years in Health. They had teamed up on the legislation to provide for abortion services following the referendum to repeal the Eighth Amendment. They had clashed on the CervicalCheck controversy. Harris had publicly aligned himself with patient advocates such as Vicky Phelan, Lorraine Walsh and Stephen Teap, while Holohan had been heavily criticized. Things did improve between the Minister and the Chief Medical Officer, though almost out of necessity. 'They didn't have a very good relationship throughout Simon Harris's tenure,' says one Department of Health official. 'It changed then. They were grand, they got on well. Once Covid arrived, they had to dig down in the trenches together.'

By the time Simon Harris was back in the Department, and his colleagues at Government were safely back in theirs, the running of the Covid show was already in full swing. 'By the time they got back,' says one senior official, 'and realized there was something going on here that they needed to turn their attention to, other than their own elections, we were up and running.'

NPHET had already conducted a number of meetings. Dr Tony Holohan and his deputy Dr Ronan Glynn were already giving interviews to the national media. The caretaker administration was content to let the civil servants and health advisers carry on.

On the first day TDs returned to Leinster House, Ronan Glynn had organized a briefing for people in the political sphere who were returning to work on the national level to try to bring them up to speed on the growing risk associated with the coronavirus. The meeting was held in Buswells Hotel, across the street from Leinster House, a familiar haunt for lunching politicians and staffers and also a venue for lobby groups and NGOs to hold launches that could draw in politicos. Glynn sat downstairs in the briefing room. He noted that two people attended the meeting, neither of them elected representatives. 'I fully understand why there were very few people there,' he says, 'but equally it shows that even at that point, it still hadn't captured broader attention.'

A week later, the conversation was growing. The blindfold of blissful innocence was coming off. Glynn held a second briefing, this time in the Audio-Visual Room of Leinster House 2000, the modern annexe of the Dáil. This time, about twenty people attended, dotted around the tiered benches of the AV Room's small lecture hall set-up. There were perhaps 'a handful' of politicians in the audience, according to one of them: Micheál Martin, leader of Fianna Fáil. Martin had some experience in public health, having served as the Minister for Health

11

during the SARS scare, navigating a tricky situation in 2003 when the WHO criticized his move to ban teams from affected countries from travelling to Ireland for the Special Olympics. Martin was caught between a rock and a hard place then, with Taoiseach Bertie Ahern on the receiving end of proddings from the Kennedy dynasty urging Ireland to let the games go ahead. During that time, Martin worked with Dr Tony Holohan, then serving as Deputy CMO. Now, with a new spectre on the horizon, Martin was curious. He tapped his feet, scribbled notes and, to some eye-rolling and at least one sigh of 'here we go' among other attendees, reminded the captive audience about his own SARS experience. He asked about asymptomatic transmission, he says, and had mentioned his concerns about the virus on the campaign trail to younger party staff who were out canvassing with him.

If the Fianna Fáil leader, or any politician, was genuinely concerned about it, it certainly didn't feature in any of the campaigning.

Leinster House, Dublin 2, 17 February 2020

Journalists gathered in the cold and dark on the plinth in front of Leinster House. Inside, the Fine Gael parliamentary party and Taoiseach Leo Varadkar were counting the cost of an electoral defeat that saw them all but voted out of office. The mood in the party was one of resignation about the losses suffered, but determination not to enter a coalition with Fianna Fáil. They would be out of government after nine years.

There was chatter among the assembled journalists about how to spread out questions over the limited time that would likely be available to them. It had been a full-on period for the press. Casual conversations in early 2020 were about how front-loaded the news year would be. 'We're having our busiest time right now at the outset of the year. Should quieten down for a time after this.'

One journalist piped up, wondering if we should ask Varadkar about the coronavirus. There was a small amount of mirth at this comment and possibly a groan or two. If the question was asked that evening, it didn't pick up any coverage.

For Fine Gael, the feeling was that this was the beginning of the end. They would serve out their time as a caretaker government and refresh themselves on the opposition benches. The speculation and horse-trading around Leinster House about government formation would continue for weeks and months to come.

The new threat of a virus of international concern changed things between Minister Simon Harris and his CMO, but there was still friction. At NPHET's meeting on 25 February, already its eighth of the crisis to date, Simon Harris's special adviser Sarah Bardon issued an invitation to journalists to attend the opening of the meeting – which would be addressed by the minister.

Nobody, however, had told Tony Holohan, who was shocked when he saw camera crews elbowing their way into the glass conference room. Holohan, privately, fumed at Sarah Bardon and called the minister aside. He expressed the importance of the independence of NPHET. Either you can be here or I can be here, but not both of us, Holohan implied.

It was a short discussion in the corner of the briefing room but it would have long-lasting consequences. Holohan explained to Harris that the experts and advisers in the room couldn't conduct business as frankly and properly as they should if a minister was present. Perhaps they might hold something back. Perhaps they might try to impress the minister with reams of knowledge, slowing the process down. Perhaps the public might not take heed of the warnings if the membership of NPHET could be seen as politically swayed. In any case, Harris got the message quickly and agreed to leave. After a few short remarks of gratitude, he and the press pack scampered out of the room and let the meeting continue in his absence.

By late February, apprehension about the looming threat was turning to genuine concern, bordering on fear. If there were lingering hopes that the full force of this virus could be avoided, that it would be limited to China and a smattering of countries across the map, they were fading and fading fast.

The first cases in the European Union had been confirmed. Italy was where the virus had made landfall on the continent. By 22 February, five people had died there, 165 people had tested positive for Covid in Lombardy, and 50,000 people had been told to quarantine in place across eleven towns in the north of the country. Quarantine was not new to Italians; the word derives from the *quaranta giorni* (forty days) ships would be forced to anchor at port before being allowed to dock in Venice during the plague. The same cities that saw almost half of their populations wiped out in that pandemic – Bergamo, Bologna, Florence – would now be the epicentres of suffering once more.

NPHET pored over data and epidemiological reports from across the world. Dr Breda Smyth, a public health specialist at the HSE, had been co-opted onto the CMO's team. She led presentations on the early international experiences. The mortality was increasing. Early reports of the impacts on older people and the medically vulnerable were starting to filter through the noisy data. At one meeting in particular, according to attendees, 'the emotional energy of the room changed. I remember looking up and looking around the room and the faces were different. They were absolutely taken aback.' Dr Smyth herself remembers sleepless nights in those early weeks, lying in bed consumed with worry about what was coming. Often, she'd wake in the middle of the night, worrying about papers she'd read or how the virus might impact Ireland. 'A lot of this information, I didn't really share with anyone. It was too scary.' The NPHET meetings were procedural, driven by presentations and matter-of-fact interventions and suggestions. They were not driven by dramatics or sweeping statements.

At the end of Dr Smyth's presentation, after a brief pause, a sentence was uttered that 'hung in the air for what seemed like minutes', according to Aoife Gillivan, sitting in on the meeting with the Department of Health Communications cohort. 'This is going to be like nothing we've ever seen before.'

Chapter 2: Arrival

In late February, the shop windows, billboards and bus-stop ads of Ireland were turning yellow. A massive public awareness campaign was launched to warn against the risks of importing coronavirus. The Department of Health's Head of Communications, Deirdre Watters, chose yellow for the colour scheme. Yellow was a dreaded historic signifier of contagion. 'The abominable yellow flag,' as a nineteenth-century traveller, Edwin Montague, described it, 'marks our ship as "plague smitten". Every boat steers off from us, afraid of contamination.' We'll never look at the colour quite the same way again. If the virus hadn't been confirmed to have arrived yet, the panic certainly had. Supermarkets were seeing early signs of people stocking up on pasta shells, tinned soup, powdered baby milk, slabs of water bottles, hand gels and disinfectant wipes.

The 27 February edition of Joe Duffy's *LiveLine* on RTÉ Radio 1 entertained calls from members of the public pulling together pandemic survival 'kits' that included axes and rope, in case the virus led to the downfall of society as we know it. All the while, the authorities were trying to project calm.

The first major flashpoint in the official response to the pandemic came following the NPHET meeting of 25 February. At the meeting, discussion was had around the staging of the Ireland vs Italy Six Nations match at the Aviva Stadium. The situation in Italy was worsening at pace. Thousands of fans coming from the hotbed of Italian rugby in the north of the country would be a severe risk.

Simon Harris, earlier scolded for stepping into the meeting in front of the cameras, had been waiting around for it to end. He had arranged to do interviews with Virgin Media News and RTÉ following the NPHET meeting and wanted to know what was going on. When he met Holohan after the meeting, he immediately asked about the rugby.

The Minister hadn't intended to go on the national airwaves with the sole purpose of calling off the rugby match, but that's exactly what transpired. The immediate reaction was torrential. Tweets and messages were flying everywhere. From the public, including seasoned current affairs writers and presenters, the initial feeling was that this was a major overreaction to something that, at that time, many people still compared to the flu. On a more official level, there was a genuine sense of shock that the Minister for Health had made this announcement before the Irish Rugby Football Union (IRFU) had been informed.

It's understood that a senior Communications official in the Department of Health had tried to call the IRFU's Head of Communications but no connection was made. The Sports Minister, Shane Ross, who had lost his seat at the election and was one of three senior Cabinet members who were being carried along in a bewildering gust through the early days of the caretaker administration, was left with a furious IRFU to deal with. He was not informed of the move either. Neither was the Taoiseach, Leo Varadkar. 'He didn't tell me, he didn't tell anyone,' says one senior member of the Government. 'That's the way Simon operated.'

The announcement provoked considerable consternation. The following day, an IRFU delegation arrived at Miesian Plaza to meet the Health Minister. Stopping to speak to reporters on the way in, the IRFU's Philip Browne said it was very 'unfair' for the Department of Health to ask the sporting body to cancel

17

the match rather than issuing a directive. The meeting was terse but polite. It was over in a couple of minutes; then the rugby delegation was given tea and coffee and space to write a press release confirming the cancellation.

Not everyone was quite so satisfied, however. At a meeting at the Department of the Taoiseach, Leo Varadkar expressed serious frustration over the decision to call off the match. In front of a gathering that included a number of advisers, Department of Health Secretary General Jim Breslin, CMO Dr Tony Holohan and top civil servant Martin Fraser, Varadkar was vocal. 'He gave out yards,' says one person who was in the room. 'It was the first time there was any real friction between the Health side and Government, and Simon was very much taking the hit for it.' It was an uncomfortable moment, excruciatingly drawn-out, and it left nobody in the room with any doubt about the Taoiseach's view on the cancellation.

Varadkar, for his part, says he 'definitely had reservations' about calling off the match, but that it was 'the right decision' and it didn't 'annoy him'. 'I knew it was coming and I knew it was the right decision and I knew it was the one that we were making.'

One of his concerns turned out to be a very common one. In the course of the meeting, he made the point that there would be no stopping the Italian travelling fans from making the trip anyway. No directive was issued. One minister, who expressed the view to me privately at the time, says: 'I can remember thinking, "In the name of Jaysus, why are we even having a conversation about allowing Italians come over to Ireland?" Just no way. We were looking at nightly footage of military shutting down Lombardy. I couldn't understand it.'

Travel advice was very limited in late February and early March. By then, the first cases of coronavirus were already being seeded in the country. Ski trips to Italy became a major focus, particularly school tours. But the concerns had been creeping in for quite some time.

* * * *

In early February, HSE Chief Executive Paul Reid remembers waiting to hear about a suspected case of coronavirus arriving on a flight into Dublin from Moscow. It sparked a small flurry of tweets on social media at the time. The Chinese national was led off the plane by officials wearing hazmat suits.

Reid was in a bar at the time. But his mind was elsewhere. Stepping out on occasion to take calls and check in to see how the situation was progressing, Reid recalls, 'I remember having a pint, it was a Saturday night and it was in and out ... Eventually, I just said "Ah here", and went home.'

The tone from Reid and the HSE team over the month of February became more serious. 'There was a sense of impending doom but not action,' says Dr Vida Hamilton, an intensive care consultant and the HSE's National Clinical Adviser and Group Lead for Acute Hospitals.

Conversations had already been had about morgue capacity, field hospitals and more. The public messaging was around allaying any sense of panic. The risk of importation was deemed 'low', and there was 'no evidence' to suggest that wearing a mask or face covering would help to protect the public. Guidance on travel was scant. Advice had been offered to the airports since January but the only travel advisory to the public was to self-isolate for fourteen days *if* you had symptoms or had been in close contact with a coronavirus case and you had been to parts of northern Italy, China, Iran, South Korea, Singapore or Japan.

With St Patrick's Day, Cheltenham and many more tourist breaks on the horizon, the message was clear – travel was still permitted. Holohan says that any moves to shut down travel at that stage would have been 'disproportionate'. 'It's difficult to kind of say the point at which, had we known something at the time, we would have applied it. You simply just don't know things until you know them.'

* * * *

On 27 February, the first confirmed case of Covid on the island of Ireland was diagnosed. A woman travelling back from Italy with her child passed through Dublin Airport and took the Enterprise train service from Connolly Station to Belfast, where she started to display symptoms. Public health doctors in Dublin and Belfast scrambled to identify anyone who had come into prolonged close contact with the family, working with the airline and public transport operators. The following day, the Republic's first case was diagnosed.

It was a Saturday. By then, more than six hundred tests had been conducted by the NVRL on the UCD campus in Dublin. There had been three weeks of nothing. No detections whatsoever. The staff there had become jittery. Most other countries across Western Europe had by now reported a 'Detected' sample. Some worried that there might be a problem with the diagnostic assay. Without positive samples coming through, it was nearly impossible for the lab staff to know whether or not the process was working.

Dr Cillian De Gascun was out for lunch with a friend home from the United States. 'Had the results not come through, we might have had sort of a longer and boozier lunch than we otherwise did.' The phone buzzed while he was at his table. Scientist Brian Keogan, who had performed the test, was on the line: 'We have one.'

There was a strange relief to the call. The process, developed by German virologist Christian Drosten, worked. The polymerase chain reaction (PCR) test, which detects the genetic material of the virus, had come back with a 'rip-roaring positive'; the viral load was through the roof.

To be absolutely certain about this milestone, De Gascun and Keogan agreed to put the samples through a second PCR line, developed by commercial labs. De Gascun, while awaiting the second test result, made the mistake of calling Tony Holohan to tell him about the positive.

What followed was hours of nervous waiting as the lab waited for the second sample. Holohan grumbled as he called De Gascun a couple of times more, scrambling to make sure measures were in place for a press briefing to get the word out to the public.

A Department of Health communications staffer rang around their contacts to find someone to run the audio-visual system at the briefing, which would be held in the department's town hall room, soon to become a very familiar sight to households across Ireland. One turned down the request because he was booked in to do the sound at a Gavin James concert at the 3Arena.

Deirdre Watters was driving to Tipperary, on what she thought was the first day to breathe freely after six weeks of intense awareness campaign preparations. The phone rang. It was Holohan. She had just arrived in the hotel car park and didn't set foot out of the car, turning it around and heading back up the motorway towards the Department. She says she bawled her eyes out on the way back to Dublin. 'It's here now.'

John Cuddihy, interim Head of the HPSC, made his way up from Kilkenny, where he was celebrating his birthday. 'There were people in his house for his party,' sympathizes Cillian De Gascun, 'and he left and I don't think he got back to Kilkenny for about two weeks afterwards.'

The pressure was on. Whisperings of a confirmed case in the Republic were filtering out. Journalists were pushing to get the story. The person at the centre of the case was a student at

Scoil Chaitríona in Glasnevin, Dublin. He had recently returned from a skiing trip in northern Italy. For the Health insiders, the focus was on contact tracing, informing the person's family and working on a response to issue to the school.

With the case confirmed, a pack of journalists crowded into the Department of Health at 9.30 p.m. for the press briefing, the first of what would become daily media appearances by the CMO. They sat clumped together, weeks still before social distancing became the done thing. Some chatted nervously, others shifted in their seats and refreshed their Twitter feeds in silence.

The Department initially did not want the school's name to be mentioned for fear it would spook people from coming forward with symptoms in the future. A letter from the local HSE Public Health department to staff and parents of students at the school, informing them of a two-week closure, was widely shared on social media and sparked a furore as to whether or not the details should be made public.

Dr Ronan Glynn, who flanked Holohan at that press conference, looks back on that briefing as being one of high tension. 'I've seen images of it; the three of us at the table look worried. What I remember about that press conference was the quietness of the room. The journalists were worried.'

Holohan himself made something of a slip in the course of the press conference. After being asked by Virgin Media News's Zara King about the measures being introduced to protect staff and students at the unnamed school, the Chief Medical Officer mentioned that it was an 'individual child' who had been infected, before denying having said it.

The Taoiseach's phone beeped with a text notification from Simon Harris: 'Call me when you can.' Varadkar asked him straight out, 'You're going to tell me we've had our first Covid case, aren't you?'

Varadkar is critical of the early advice given by NPHET. It's one thing that members of NPHET say in hindsight they would change. There was a lag in reaching decisions on key issues like Cheltenham, on which no advice was given for returnees unless they had developed symptoms, or the St Patrick's Day parades until a week before they would have been held. 'The strategy was slow,' Varadkar says. 'Herd immunity was never our strategy but the strategy was slow. The advice from Tony and co. wasn't "Shut down the country immediately and don't let any cases in," which potentially maybe we should have done.'

He notes that the advice from the European Centre for Disease Prevention and Control (ECDC) and the WHO was not to unnecessarily disrupt international travel. 'The official advice was that cancelling St Patrick's Day was excessive. So, you know, it's gone over and back but actually, weirdly at the start, it was the politicians who were taking the more action-driven approach.'

NPHET was finding its feet at press briefings and tried to explain complex matters to a nervous public, which was undergoing a crash course in epidemiology. R numbers, community transmission, PCRs were all absorbed with the concentration of a student cramming for exams. The explanations weren't always pristine.

In early March, minutes before a press conference, Dr Ronan Glynn had a brainwave. As the public health experts struggled to explain what was and what wasn't considered close contact, Glynn piped up. 'Maybe I could do a diagram.' He began to doodle on an easel in the boardroom, but there was no time to practise. 'Great, just do that.' Journalists waiting in the briefing room were told to expect a visual aid to help parents to understand contacts and 'contacts of contacts' in schools, and a whiteboard appeared alongside the top table. I shuffled to the front row of seats, to get a good vantage point to video it for Twitter, hoping for a useful, shareable video that would prove revelatory.

Glynn began his presentation, his green marker squeaking

awkwardly in a deathly silence. When he turned to face his audience, a stick figure had appeared on the board beside him. He was met by a sea of grimaces and was instantly mortified. He worried it would become a meme. A stick figure would not reassure a frightened nation.

Days later, he would conduct his first live television interview with me on Virgin Media. In the minutes before we went live, he shifted his feet, wiped the sweat from his brow and asked where he should look. His voice trembled a little, his nerves obvious. Glynn was learning communications on the fly and it didn't come naturally to him.

From Lydican in Oranmore, County Galway, Glynn's parents run Glynn's Fruit and Veg, a family business for more than 85 years whose logo still takes pride of place on Claregalway's GAA jersey. He trained initially as a physio, graduating in 2002, before training as a doctor in Scotland. Little over a year into his position as Deputy CMO, the softly spoken and genial Glynn had not yet turned forty and had been blasted into a position of key leadership in a national emergency. He would have to learn fast. There were bigger tests to come.

Cases continued to materialize over the days ahead. First another case, then four more – a family from County Clare, which resulted in the closure of three schools with over seven hundred contacts; then seven more on 5 March.

It was on this day that fears began to escalate significantly in the medical community. One of those seven cases was confirmed as the first case of community transmission – there was no known link to travel to northern Italy, or contact with an already confirmed case. The patient, a forty-three-year-old farmer, had been on a trolley in Cork University Hospital (CUH). The hospital immediately kicked into overdrive. It was an evening of high drama. Journalists were being called by frightened medics in Cork. Their colleagues across the country were on high alert too. The patient in question may have been infectious and had been in close contact with staff members and patients for days.

The patient was treated by Dr Corinna Sadlier. Her suspicions had been raised by his pneumonia-like symptoms. 'I wonder,' she thought, 'if this could be SARS-CoV-2.' She persisted, even though there was no known travel link, in seeking a test. Her colleague, infectious diseases consultant Professor Mary Horgan, believes it was one of the first times when medical instinct had played a key role in the management of the virus. 'It isn't always based on protocols and "you have to go by the book all the time", it's your gut feeling,' she says.

The patient had been admitted to CUH on 25 February with a headache and an incidental cough – before the first case in the country had been confirmed. In the Emergency Department, Professor Conor Deasy said, all the preparations had been geared towards a patient coming back from China or Italy. Signs were up at the entrances to the hospital, people were screened for respiratory symptoms. The man in question came in and was placed on a hospital corridor with 'probably forty other patients', Deasy remembers. 'He was on our corridor for, I'd say, around twenty-four hours. Then he went upstairs to MSSU, another open-plan medical ward. He spent up to thirty-six hours there.'

The man got sicker and sicker. Ultimately, on Dr Sadlier's insistence, he was swabbed. 'It opened a whole can of worms,' says Deasy. Sixty staff went into self-isolation immediately. About 780 people in total were eventually traced as casual contacts. 'We had about three hundred patients who would have been exposed ... patients, staff ... who then have to be contacted and were considered close contacts by definition.'

The patient himself was admitted to ICU and ventilated before being transferred to the Mater Hospital in Dublin, where he received specialist treatment. He died in April.

The admission of the first case of community transmission

was the first 'red alert' moment for authorities. There was now a live possibility of widespread transmission of the virus in the community. Rumours and panic spread like wildfire the night the case was diagnosed by CUH. At home in Dublin 15, my phone buzzed with messages from isolating medics in CUH and their concerned colleagues across Ireland sounding the alarm. Some of the messages urged me to run down to the supermarket and stock up on essentials and warn my in-laws in West Cork that they'd need to stay indoors for days to come.

Testing capacity, soon to become a major focus of the State's response, was also coming more into the spotlight. 'Capacity might have been an issue,' says the NVRL's Cillian De Gascun, 'but obviously we still had the requirement for travel as an indication for testing at that stage. Whereas, you know, you could argue we should have lifted that sooner.'

Travel continued for symptomless arrivals for weeks to come, and until well into March testing continued to be determined by whether or not someone had travelled to an at-risk area.

* * * *

The once-sleepy Tyrolean village of Ischgl in Austria's Paznaun Valley was now anything but. It became popular with skiers from Germany, the Netherlands and Italy in the 1980s and has since exploded in popularity with tourists from Ireland and the UK. It's been marketed as the Ibiza of the Alps. '*Relax. If you can ...*' has become the resort's party-driven slogan after a rebranding campaign that has seen it take on a glam rock-style logo and play host to massive mountaintop concerts by international superstars like Elton John, Rihanna, Muse and Pink.

Some local bars thrive on the reputation of *Wahnsinn*, German for 'craziness', with thumping music all night, cheap schnapps, beer and shots keeping punters going until the wee hours and beyond. As a destination, it is difficult to match.

Tens of thousands of ski boots thump through the village every year, with forty-five ski lifts linking the centre of the village with over two hundred kilometres of slopes.

But in the early days of spring 2020, it was no paradise. It became a 'ground zero' of infection for Europe, marked out as one of the continent's first super-spreader events that caught unknowing, unfortunate holidaymakers from Ireland in its midst while authorities and the town cottoned on too late to a disaster in the making.

On 29 February, hairdresser Eóin Wright from Kilmainham, Dublin, was at the airport. The laughter had already started and it wouldn't stop until he and his group of six friends got back in a week's time. The lads had been going to Ischgl for about fifteen years now. They'd befriended Mario, a local ski instructor, who ran a small *pension* guesthouse. He'd flown to Dublin a few times and effectively became a family friend to each of them. That evening, the Republic would confirm its first case of Covid, but there was no travel guidance issued for Austria; the focus of health authorities across Europe was solely across the Alps in northern Italy.

Eóin's wife, he says, is something of a 'Covid policewoman'. She had warned that perhaps he should give it a miss this year; she had a nagging worry in the back of her mind that he might catch this new virus on his trip. Eóin and his friends weren't putting a stop to their travels now, however; as far as they were concerned, there was no reason to. There were no local reports of any major Covid issues.

That same day, another group of five Irish skiers were also flying out. Speaking under condition of anonymity, *Barry*, from the south of the country, and his four friends had been in Ischgl several times before. The flight that morning was full. The majority of the people on the plane, in their bright puffer jackets, were certainly going skiing. When they arrived, there was no sense of a catastrophe brewing. The slopes were pure, the skies were bright blue and things were just heavenly. At night, the bars were busy.

'When I say they were jam-packed, they were shoulder to shoulder,' says Barry, who had to battle through the heaving crowds, drenched in sweat, to get to one bar as the sounds of 'crappy German europop' music made it a battle to be heard even when shouting at the top of your voice. Staff used whistles to try to get through the throngs.

'It's every Irish bar at Christmas,' is Eóin's description of Ischgl's aprés ski scene. Eóin felt he missed some of what's been written in the months since – scenes of people dancing on tables and having shots poured into their mouths passed him by – and he laughs: 'Shit, how did I miss out on that?'

On the Wednesday night, members of both Barry and Eoin's parties went into Kitzloch, a bar/restaurant with roaring fires, some of the best food in town and more than enough drink to keep thirsty skiers refreshed. The week continued as planned, both groups enjoying the skiing, with only the most cursory conversations about coronavirus. Nothing on the local television channels. No concerns raised at local bars.

While all this was happening, Iceland had raised the alarm. Skiers returning from Ischgl had tested positive for the virus. On 4 March, Iceland had designated Ischgl a 'High Risk' hotspot, on the same level as China and northern Italy.

Not a whole lot changed in Ischgl. Skiing and travelling parties continued until 13 March. The Irish groups of Barry and Eóin left on the changeover day of Saturday 7 March. Eóin and the lads said goodbye to Mario, their host, and were already looking forward to the next trip.

On that day, a thirty-six-year-old barman at Kitzloch, where both Irish groups had been on the Wednesday, became the first person to test positive for Covid in the village itself. On the Friday night, the deputy head of the Tyrol Chamber of Commerce, Franz Hörl, sent a text message to the owner of the

Kitzloch bar. The text, leaked to the Austrian news site Kurier, urged him to shut his bar down or he would be to blame for ending the season in Ischgl and possibly Tyrol. A second text, mere minutes later, told him the eyes of the country were on the bar. Kitzloch shut. If Ischgl had shut down at the same time, critics say, thousands of infections could have been prevented.

By the time the Irish travellers arrived home, Covid was a much bigger story than when they left. Eóin was mindful of this. He called the HSE helpline, telling them his group had come back from skiing in Austria and asking for guidance. 'No, no,' he says the helpline told him. 'Continue on.' So they did.

Two days later, the phone rang. It was Mario. He warned him about the news from Kitzloch. Eóin called his friend Dave Coffey, a GP, and asked for his advice. Dave told him to play it safe and stay at home for the next few days. Eóin, even though it was a busy time in the salon with the bank holiday weekend approaching, was minded to do the right thing and take no risks. A few days later, 'the shit hit the fan', he says. Clusters had started to emerge across the continent: in Germany, Sweden, Denmark and Norway – all among holidaymakers returning from the resort.

One of Eóin's group had started to feel unwell and tested positive for Covid. By the Saturday, Eóin himself was feeling unwell. He had been in work the two days after returning from Ischgl and was immediately concerned for his staff and customers. Twelve staff in the salon and twenty customers had to be tested. Their results all came up as 'Not Detected', a huge relief to Eóin, who could now focus on his own situation.

In the south, the notification ding from Barry's WhatsApp group with his four mates was the sound of trouble. One of the party had felt unwell and had requested a Covid test. He tested positive on the Wednesday. Barry got tested and went into isolation while he waited for his result. 'It wasn't much fun. Netflix got a good rattle.'

Of the eleven people across both parties, all tested positive for Covid-19. Eóin Wright subsequently suffered the impacts of loss of taste and smell for over a year.

The international focus on Ischgl has been intense. An independent investigation found 'momentous' errors in how local authorities reacted. World news media compared the resort's slow response with that of the mayor of Amity Island in *Jaws*, headlines blaring 'Everyone was drenched in the virus.' On the continent, a major class action lawsuit has been launched by the Austrian consumer lawyer Peter Kolba. More than six thousand people have joined the lawsuit from forty-five countries, including Ireland. Thousands of cases across Europe resulted from a two-week period in Ischgl. The Irish groups, despite their diagnoses, say that they don't blame Ischgl for the outbreaks. 'I'd go back in the morning,' says Barry. 'And I will go back. I guarantee it.'

'Relax. If you can …' Ischgl's slogan isn't quite so alluring now.

Chapter 3: The Gathering Storm

The Sycamore Room, Government Buildings,
Monday, 9 March 2020

'You're not relieved of your duty just yet, I'm afraid,' chuckled Leo Varadkar. 'We may need you for a few more weeks or months yet.'

Varadkar's joke across the table, aimed at Regina Doherty, Minister for Social Protection, was picked up by the cameras allowed into the first meeting of the Cabinet Covid Sub-Committee before they were swiftly hurried out by the minders from Government Information Services. Doherty had lost her seat in the election and she was, in her own words, 'feeling a bit sorry for myself'. She wasn't alone.

It was a strange atmosphere. Many members were still licking their wounds after the election, feeling like imposters at the top table; others were hoping to quickly run down the clock on the remaining days in their respective departments.

The ministers battled for space, elbow to elbow in a crisis meeting that would prolong their stay in the prime real estate of office. Jackets were flung over the backs of chairs, and the smell of bad coffee was pungent. Paschal Donohoe was locked in conversation with Simon Coveney, Fine Gael's Brexit double act back together but yet to fully appreciate the economic disaster soon to be laid bare. Varadkar beamed as he was flanked by his two most trusted advisers, Brian Murphy and Martin Fraser, the most powerful 'mandarin' in the country. Simon Harris, in shirtsleeves, sipped from his reusable water bottle and wedged himself between Donohoe and Tony Holohan, who exchanged brief pleasantries with Paul Reid of the HSE, battle lines between them yet to be drawn. At the far end of the table, Robert Watt, the hawkish Secretary General at the Department of Public Expenditure and Reform, bounced his pen on his notes, appearing stony-faced as the camera shutters snapped.

As the meeting began, tension set in. Snapping the legs of his eyeglasses shut, Holohan went through the projections on the monitor at the head of the table. The projections put forward by Holohan and Paul Reid at the briefing stunned everyone: 1.9 million people in Ireland could get sick; somewhere between 25,000 and 35,000 people could die if action wasn't taken.

Finance Minister Donohoe was floored. 'It was terrible. Discussions began about "if a certain number of people die, how would we cope with that?"' The scale of the effort that would be required to shore up Ireland's defences was immense.

The challenges that would test them were monstrous.

'We began to realize how quickly we would need to scale up our hospitals and began to realize that even if we did absolutely everything that we needed to do, it mightn't be enough,' says Donohoe. 'Or we mightn't be able to get there quickly enough.' He was reeling. 'You're thinking "What if?" We had so much to do, so quickly, with this awful challenge and this awful sinking feeling that it just might not be enough.'

The room froze. Ministers and senior civil servants were silent, horrified by what was by now playing out in Italy and what could soon be arriving on Ireland's shores in numbers that could lead to the deaths of tens of thousands of people.

'There's little that can prepare you for being in a room and you're being told that thousands of people could die.

Thousands. And this could be one of those moments in which you're talking about how all you can do is reduce the loss of life,' says one senior minister, still shaken by the memory.

Varadkar, noting months later that the modelling was 'way out', said privately to his advisers that if Ireland could manage to keep deaths under 20,000, 'we'll have done really well.' Others, like Simon Harris, hit back at this notion, saying that some people 'sneeringly' hitting out at the modelling should realize that it was predicated on there being no State interventions or restrictions.

The Taoiseach was instantly taken by the graph on intensive care units (ICUs), stunned by how quickly capacity would be reached. As a doctor, he knew what happens when you go beyond that point. Treating ICU patients outside ICU; the ethical dilemmas that would arise – 'Doctors having to do the one thing you hate to do, which is to choose who to ventilate and who to not.' There was, however, a peculiar freedom in the Taoiseach's mind. Leo Varadkar found himself untethered from the normal constraints of politics. 'No need to worry about opinion polls or interest groups or elections,' he says, 'that was all out of the way.'

At the meeting, the decision was taken, finally, after weeks of speculation, to cancel the St Patrick's Day festival, now just one week away. There had been pushback to that decision in the run-up to the Cabinet sub-committee meeting. Simon Harris, among others, was vocally calling for it, simply not understanding the hold-up. Others, like Paschal Donohoe and Robert Watt, were very concerned with the economic impact of lost revenue from one of the busiest weekends on the tourism calendar.

As one senior minister put it: 'There are some people in this country – and some of them are politicians – who have a tendency to think that places like the Department of Health overreact. "Who are those Puritans over there in

33

Health? What are they at now? What's wrong with a bit of rugby or a St Patrick's Day? Should we not do what they did in Sweden?"' referring to the 'hands off' approach of the Swedish government.

While the big decisions were made at the sub-committee, ministers who weren't involved were rankled. The likes of agriculture minister Michael Creed and rural development minister Michael Ring railed against the sense that politics was slowly being consumed by civil servants and public health officials. Martin Fraser, described by some as the sixteenth member of the Cabinet, was becoming increasingly critical to the running of the show.

'His voice was the most influential one at the table,' says one minister. 'He was untouchable'.

Fraser would cajole the ministers who wavered on the need for quick action, metaphorically banging heads together. 'Listen, you're not in the real world, lads. This is a serious disease. There's no time for messing around.'

'He's brilliant and a bollocks,' says one minister. 'He is brilliant at getting shit done. He's worked his way up and he's a grafter. But he's coarse [...] he'd bollock people out a bit too much for my liking in front of other people.'

These included ministers. And, in the time to come, the CMO.

Department of Health, Wednesday, 11 March 2020

'Oh fuck!'

'What?'

Cillian De Gascun's phone screen flashed with a text from his colleagues at the National Virus Reference Laboratory.

'There are twenty positives.'

The Director of the NVRL was debriefing with Tony Holohan

and Ronan Glynn after another lengthy press conference. The message on De Gascun's phone would change everything. Glynn and Holohan looked at each other in shock.

In a day, Ireland effectively saw its caseload double. That night, the Republic recorded its first death from the virus. An older woman had died in Naas General Hospital in County Kildare. It was instantly clear to the officials in the room that action would be needed. Holohan took the lead: 'Okay, we need a NPHET meeting this evening – 9.15 p.m.'

The texts and phone calls began. A member of the communications team was dispatched across the street to Chai Yo to fetch a mountain of Chinese food for the arriving officials. Ahead of a meeting that would prove to be a turning point in the recent history of the State, Tony Holohan and his NPHET colleagues were sitting and waiting. 'I don't think we necessarily knew where the meeting was going to end up,' remembers Cillian De Gascun.

Holohan called the minister. Harris was at home cooking dinner. He knew the Chief Medical Officer was very worried. When the call came about the emergency meeting, Harris headed straight from Greystones back to the Department, stopping to text the Taoiseach, who was in Washington, DC for St Patrick's Day and phoning Varadkar's chief of staff, Brian Murphy, and Tánaiste Simon Coveney.

'I need you to come into Health, serious things are happening,' he told Coveney. The Tánaiste had been working late and was getting settled in his Dublin apartment when the call came through. With Varadkar abroad in Washington, Harris needed a senior member of Government in tow to take leadership. Both Simons arrived at Miesian Plaza after 9 p.m., just as the NPHET meeting was convening. Word reached the meeting that the Tánaiste had arrived. More than one attendee paused to wonder, 'What the hell is he doing here?'

The meeting went on for hours. The ECDC had put together

a framework for governments on possible measures for restrictions – shutting schools, cutting down mass gatherings. This was the basis on which NPHET put together its recommendations. It was slow work. At one point, Dr Ronan Glynn looked up and scanned the meeting room. Everyone was exhausted. The low hum of office lights lit up the room, bringing into sharp relief the bags under people's eyes as they worked on recommendations that would alter the fabric of Irish life for months to come.

In a boardroom down the hall from the NPHET meeting, the two ministers waited. They were joined by the HSE CEO, Paul Reid, the Department's Secretary General Jim Breslin, Liz Canavan from the Taoiseach's department, Coveney's adviser Chris Donoghue and Harris's adviser Sarah Bardon. This gathering had been cobbled together at short notice, and they had little to do but make small talk while decisions that would instantly change the course of the country were being made a few doors down. The atmosphere was described as a bit 'doolally'. With all remaining food in the Department gone at that late hour, Sarah Bardon set off to the sixth floor looking for provisions and returned after scavenging a box of Maltesers. Simon Coveney compared the atmosphere to some of the nights of brinkmanship in Brexit negotiations. Paul Reid was in and out of the room making worried calls with HSE leadership and stepping out for tense conversations with Jim Breslin, anxious to hear about the decisions that his team would have to implement based on recommendations from Tony Holohan.

From the boardrooms, overlooking the city, you can see as far out as the airport, you can see the Aviva Stadium, you can look out to St Vincent's Hospital, back across the Northside to the Mater and beyond. Harris spent time looking out the windows and trying to imagine the people going to bed that night who had no idea what was coming for them the next morning.

The impatient table-tapping, tea-supping and chair-swivelling was halted when Holohan arrived. It was now after one in the morning. Flanked by Tracey Conroy and Fergal Goodman, his Department of Health colleagues responsible for acute hospitals and primary care respectively, Holohan produced a single sheet of paper for the minister with a number of requests.

It called for the closure of schools, childcare and higher education; offices to move to working from home wherever possible; the closure of museums, galleries and tourism sites; limiting mass gatherings to one hundred people indoors and five hundred outdoors; elderly or medically vulnerable people to reduce their contacts outside the home as much as possible; individuals to reduce their discretionary contacts as much as possible; and anyone with symptoms to self-isolate for fourteen days. Ireland was moving to the Delay phase. In truth, as many people there were aware, there was no delaying what had already arrived. There was no dissent from the ministers or from the officials. Everyone in the room had the sense that 'we were doing the right thing'.

He might have looked authoritative to the two Simons and the assortment of officials, but Holohan was tired. 'I'd left nothing on the pitch,' he says. He entered the meeting knowing that this was beyond anything he'd encountered in his career to date. Telling the Health Minister and the 'effective leader of the country', Simon Coveney, to close schools and regulate hospital visits was something that required moral support. 'I needed a bit of steel in my backbone,' he says. That's why he had picked two of his closest confidantes and colleagues, Conroy and Goodman, for extra moral support in that moment.

Liz Canavan was in contact with the Taoiseach's delegation in Washington. There was frustration in this unprecedented moment, one of the first of many in the coming days, that the head of Government was disconnected from decision-making back in Ireland. There had been thought given to calling off the Washington trip, which instead was pared back. It boiled down to the question of 'Do we stand President Trump up or not?' Varadkar was brushing shoulders with tycoons and politicians in an emerald green bow tie, and getting set for his Oval Office bilateral.

The meeting at the Department of Health finished after two in the morning as heads started to droop and ties were loosened. Simon Coveney thanked the public health officials for their work, urging them to go home and get some sleep. They stepped out into the night and didn't know what to do with themselves. There was no small talk, just a sense that the world was a very different place from the one they lived in just six hours ago. People were frightened. Cillian De Gascun, walking out to his car on Baggot Street, texted a friend in the US who he knew would be awake, just to have someone to talk to. Breda Smyth felt it was an acceptance of the inevitable, Ireland was 'hostage' to the virus until such time as a vaccine could be produced. There was no telling how long, if ever, that would be.

They'd need to be fully rested for the days ahead. Coveney's and Harris's teams would reconvene at six o'clock the following morning. Holohan left the Department after 3 a.m., jumping into a taxi, frustrated that he wouldn't get a morning walk in. 'It was one hell of a night. One hell of a night.'

* * * *

National Building Museum, Washington, DC,
Wednesday, 11 March 2020

Leo Varadkar had been enjoying his evening. The Taoiseach was getting the hang of the novel practice of fist-bumping or elbow-tapping in place of handshakes that had just started, even if some of the American hosts hadn't. One member of Varadkar's entourage repeatedly told prominent dignitaries, 'I don't meant to be rude, but I am not shaking your hand.'

The Ireland Funds Gala was an illustrious occasion, topped off with a $1,000 per plate dinner. Congressmen and women, senators, Speaker Nancy Pelosi and business magnates from across America were milling about among the magnificent Corinthian columns of the National Building Museum, among the tallest in the world, which supported a spectacular ceiling of metal and glass. The atmosphere of the grand occasion would soon be shattered.

Martin Fraser tapped Varadkar on the shoulder. 'We need to leave,' he said. 'I need to talk to you about what's happening in Dublin.' Varadkar attracted criticism in his time as Taoiseach for drawing on references to pop culture. Infamously, on meeting Theresa May in Downing Street for the first time, at a crunch point in Brexit, he giddily remarked that he was reminded of the scene in rom-com *Love Actually* where Hugh Grant's Prime Minister dad-dances up and down the staircases. Varadkar himself describes the moment he heard of the recommendations from NPHET as 'one of those kinds of scenes from a movie. Most of the time being a politician is just a normal job. You go to your meetings, you do your week, you do your paperwork, you sign your documents … Every now and then, it feels like you're the president or the prime minister from the movies.'

Varadkar was ushered through the bowels of the venue to escape upstairs and take a briefing on what was happening. The urgency of the departure caught the Irish journalists in the travelling party off-guard. They assumed Varadkar was to be briefed about the Trump administration's travel ban on arrivals from Europe, which had been announced to a flurry of screen pop-ups and murmurs at tables at the Funds dinner.

The journalists scampered after the Taoiseach, leaving their dinners behind them to race down the marble corridors to try to catch him. Aoife Grace Moore, political correspondent with the *Irish Examiner*, was one of them. 'We were yelling out "Taoiseach! Taoiseach!" Not only to get lines from him about what Trump had done but, honestly, to figure out how are we going to get out of the country.'

'When I know something, you'll know something,' the Taoiseach's press adviser Sarah Meade told the group, who were left catching their breath.

Tánaiste Simon Coveney, effectively acting as the leader of the country back in Dublin, called the Taoiseach. Varadkar, who was playing catch-up, peppered his number two with questions. There was an element, according to informed sources, of 'I left you in charge for a few days and where are we now?'

But the Government knew this was coming; Varadkar had felt it would be perhaps a week down the line, after St Patrick's Day. Martin Fraser assessed the situation and decided it was important that news of the restrictions was announced by the Taoiseach. 'Get a speech together and we'll organize a press conference.'

Varadkar headed for bed. One of the most significant speeches ever to be delivered by an Irish Taoiseach was drafted by Leo Varadkar tapping away on his iPhone screen in a guest suite at Blair House, the US President's assigned residence for visiting dignitaries and heads of state. The Taoiseach had left his laptop in Dublin. The important thing, he felt, in this speech was to balance the gravity of the situation with offering hope.

The Taoiseach finished his draft sometime after 2 a.m. Washington time. He had kept it brief. Martin Fraser, Chief of Staff Brian Murphy and Sarah Meade were up even later, putting shape on a speech that would have been beyond conception to anyone just days earlier.

A press note was texted to the travelling delegation of journalists. 'Press announcement. Blair House. 7 a.m.'

The journalists, exhausted and sleepless, hurried into position. It was still dark, and the lighting was terrible. The creased Irish tricolour beside the podium was slightly off-balance, propped up by a folded piece of cardboard. Members of the press quietly griped to each other about how tired they were. They had this unannounced stop added to the day, with the Oval Office meeting with Trump to follow. RTÉ and Virgin Media interrupted normal programming to broadcast the Taoiseach's speech.

Back in Dublin, journalists who had been told to gather for a press conference with the Tánaiste, Minister for Health and Chief Medical Officer huddled around cracked phone screens in the courtyard of Government Buildings to watch Varadkar's remarks.

'I need to speak to you about the coronavirus and Covid-19 ...'

* * * *

The morning of 12 March is one people working in politics and health will always remember. There were very clearly murmurings that something major was happening. Cabinet members, like Minister for Social Protection Regina Doherty, were sitting at home when the phone calls and texts started to come in.

'Simon Coveney rang me that morning and said "Get your make-up on and get into town early,"' she says. 'He said, "I can't tell you what's going on but you need to get into town early."' Doherty was at the counter in her kitchen with her husband, having a cup of tea.

'Shit, there's something really wrong,' she told her husband, as she grabbed her keys and coat and made for the door. Racing through her mind was a discussion on the radio the previous

41

weekend in which Professor Sam McConkey had spelled out the most grim of forecasts regarding loss of life, more than Doherty could possibly imagine. McConkey had said that between 80,000 and 120,000 lives could be lost. His projections caused massive consternation among health officials, who shook their heads and switched off radios when he came on. They were very much in a 'don't panic' mode.

There would be no Cabinet meeting before the restrictions were announced. 'We should have had,' says Varadkar. 'I sort of seized powers that are really powers for the Government rather than the Taoiseach.'

Varadkar himself was already on to the next engagement, joining Donald Trump in front of the bowl of shamrock. Irish journalists battled for prime position in a crowded room, leaning over each other, breathing down each other's necks to get microphones in front of the President and blurt questions at him. In the office of the most powerful man in the world, the smell of BO was overpowering, according to Aoife Grace Moore. 'We were all lying on top of each other. Everyone was wearing suits. Everyone was sweating on each other. Everyone.'

The Irish delegation sat on the golden sofas of the Oval Office. Martin Fraser, for once caught on camera, looked around the room observing the mayhem as Trump's handlers barked orders at the journalists. He was wedged uncomfortably between Brian Murphy and Dan Mulhall, the Irish Ambassador, with a toy plane – a model of Trump's redesigned Air Force One – sitting directly, absurdly, on a table in front of them.

At times during their broadcast remarks, Leo Varadkar's body language betrayed his nerves and the exhaustion of the last twenty-four hours. His sock had slid down his leg, revealing an awkward glimpse of calf. His eyes, pallid and gaunt, widened as Trump said the virus would 'go away' quickly, and he smiled awkwardly as the hacks were herded out of the office. Opting against the handshake, the two leaders went for a 'Namaste' greeting, a slight bow, no contact, hands together like a child's communion pose. 'It feels like you're being rude,' said Varadkar, 'but you just can't afford to think like that for the next few weeks.' *Weeks.*

The announcement of the first restrictions from both Washington and Dublin was a seminal moment. Despite the pleas of Minister Heather Humphreys from her podium in the Italian Room in Government Buildings, large queues were forming in supermarkets across the country. It was chaos. Tesco in Clarehall on Dublin's Northside closed for a time after it was overwhelmed with customers.

Social media and news items told Irish audiences that there had been a shortage of toilet paper in Australia after masses of people stockpiled vital supplies. It prompted similar moves here. Bemused gardaí in units across the country were dispatched to keep an eye on developments on supermarket aisles. WhatsApp groups all around the nation were swamped with forwarded videos of thronged Aldis and Lidls. The viral footage only drove more panic-buying.

The Government and the HSE would soon be embarking on a panic-buying spree of their own.

* * * *

'There is a lot of modern-day piracy going on … What I actually mean is, whether it's for PPE, ventilators, reagents, as soon as you think you have a stock secured … somebody, somewhere in the world is outbidding you. Whether it's at the delivery stage or it's nearly at the export stage.' HSE CEO Paul Reid wasn't hiding his frustration any longer. The battle for PPE around the world had become ferocious.

'There were countries robbing off each other and diverting flights. The idea that there was a unified global response or even a unified EU response was nonsense. It was every country for itself,' says Dr Colm Henry.

The early days of the pandemic response around the world were characterized as an out-and-out brawl between countries and health services for 'gold dust' PPE supplies. Ireland couldn't rely on Europe in this regard either. 'Europe just completely failed,' says one official, with knowledge of talks on a Union level. There was no coordination. There was no help coming from the continent. It was a free-for-all.

Ireland was alone.

This chilling isolation came to light relatively early in the pandemic. HSE procurement teams were brought together on a call by Sean Bresnan, the National Director of Procurement, an affable man ready to lead a charm offensive of the HSE's traditional supply lines. 'It was a call really to put on the green jersey.' Bresnan explained what hospitals, GPs and frontline carers would need. It became apparent very soon after that call that the traditional supply lines were 'not going to work'. 'Sorry, we can't help' was a regular response in emails and calls. This was a dark place. 'Absolute despair' is how Bresnan describes it. Plan A was already blown out of the water. Plans B, C and D would need to be written and enacted or else Ireland could face a near unmitigated spread of the virus with little protection.

Ministers pored over the details. Reid pleaded with the Cabinet for support at briefings. How much would you need? How much would it cost? Some stern letters made their way from the Department of Public Expenditure and Reform (DPER) to the Health Minister querying the spend to date. The Secretary General of DPER, Robert Watt, and Paul Reid of the HSE went back a long way. They had worked together in the Department for years during the economic recovery. Reid was forced to make the case to his old friend. 'I'd rather be looking at it than looking for it.'

As the virus gripped the country, reports of shortages became commonplace. Even hospitals like St James's, the largest in the country, had senior staff launching appeals on social media for long-sleeved gowns. The situation was dire. In mid-March, the Irish Hospital Consultants Association wrote to the Minister for Health expressing serious concerns about the lack of protective gear – stocks were 'running out' and frontline staff and the patients in their care were in 'extremely exposed positions'. Respirator masks were in short supply, goggles with poor seals fogged up quickly, some gowns tore quickly, leaving staff frightened of exposure. 'That was just a bad situation,' says one government minister. 'There's no one trying to spin our way out of that. It was horrific.'

While reports of PPE shortages were widely covered and the subject of intense scrutiny, the public did not know how close Ireland came to an unmitigated collapse of stocks. 'To be honest with you, it's probably important that they didn't,' says Professor Martin Cormican, the HSE's clinical lead on infection control. The HSE was, to his mind, being honest about how hard it was to secure new equipment, but management didn't want staff to know just how close things were to the cliff edge. 'We certainly weren't looking to draw people's attention to just how precarious it was,' says Cormican. 'It didn't help anyone. Our colleagues who were delivering hands-on care, they had enough to worry about … it was really important for people to feel secure enough to be able to work.'

Chief Clinical Officer Dr Colm Henry admits that Ireland came within mere 'days' of running out of PPE. Staff were forced to re-use visors. Orders of gowns came in too short. 'We were scared,' admits Paul Reid. 'Let's be frank, because the manufacturing had ceased in China.'

In the early days, the HSE was working on orders of 250,000 masks, not realizing that in effect that was only a quarter of the daily demand across the health sector. The volume of everything required was beyond any available comparison. If it was available and it could be brought in, the sentiment was that we should attempt to have it. 'It was a question of close your eyes and authorize,' says one official with knowledge of the procurement process. 'That's how it had to be. And by God, we needed it.'

Discussions at National Crisis Management Team level were grisly to an unprecedented degree. 'It was absolute fear,' says Bresnan. HSE bosses focused on how Ireland would handle mass deaths. What the bodybag capacity of the State was. Where would morgues be needed. All of this was informed by the unfolding human disaster in Italy where military vehicles were now being used to transport the dead from packed mortuaries to crematoriums.

'The first surge,' says Dr Colm Henry, 'was characterized by us groping in the dark. We were trying to buy every gun, every weapon, every defence we could get without knowing how we were going to be attacked.' Everything was in short supply. Testing capacity was a fraction of what was needed. 'Tests would take days to come back,' he says.

Trade embargoes on PPE went up across traditional markets. Countries that would otherwise be the most reliable suppliers of equipment for Irish hospitals were throwing up walls, requisitioning what they needed for their own frontlines.

Nothing that followed was simple. 'It was like flying a plane but building the plane in the air as you go,' was a description that became popular among the procurement team and the arms of the State that were involved in the effort.

On 12 March, as the first restrictions were being announced, Bresnan was arriving at the gates of the Chinese Embassy in Ballsbridge. Bresnan, along with representatives from The Department of Foreign Affairs, The Department of Enterprise and the Industrial Development Authority (IDA), was met by a security guard. The guard took a look in the car window and presented each of them with a facemask. It gave Bresnan a strange shiver. 'Jesus,' he thought. 'This is the territory we might be heading to in the months to come.'

The meeting with Ambassador He Xiangdong went well. The ambassador was receptive. The HSE's appeals were getting a hearing, at least. But there were no guarantees of success. As Bresnan walked back out onto Merrion Road, he prayed to himself that some good would come of it. If it didn't pay off, 'we'd be a hell of a lot worse off'.

News filtered through to Bresnan days later that a meeting had been secured with China Resources Pharmaceutical. Here we go. He spent the night before the teleconference on Google Translate, his face lit by his screen, scrolling for Chinese phrases he could learn off by heart. 'Happy St Patrick's Day' was one. Another was along the lines of, 'Your help, your support and your encouragement is so needed by the Irish people.' HSE members involved in the efforts remain convinced that small touches like this were key to greasing the wheel, showing respect and gratitude to the Chinese.

The deal was on; €200m worth of PPE had been tied up with China Resources. Reid and Bresnan's first, last and only hope in those days was the Chinese Ambassador. Ambassador He became personal friends with Reid. The Ambassador would call him and address the HSE chief as 'Dr Reid'. 'I'm not a doctor,' Reid would reply. 'He called me Dr Reid so I called him Dr He (pronounced phonetically as Dr Who).' The name gave the HSE team many a giggle in those dark times. In an exercise of soft power and diplomacy, Reid got the Taoiseach and the Health Minister to thank the ambassador for his assistance.

Representatives of the IDA, which already had a presence in China, were signed up to act as sourcing agents. The Defence Forces were readied to be the ground crew. Aer Lingus signed on to create an 'air bridge'. The country wanted heroes. People stuck at home, watching the evening news, needed someone to root for. This was one of those moments. As many as ninety Aer Lingus pilots volunteered for the flights, which would see five Airbuses take off from Dublin every day, land in China, take on board the massive consignments, immediately take off again and get it back home.

The jets weren't designed for this. Every seat was used to hold boxes upon boxes of masks and gowns until the plane was completely full. Strict quarantine rules meant there would be no time for pilots to open up and get some air before beginning the second leg of the twenty-eight-hour round trip. A fully laden Airbus A330 could carry about 60,000 gowns. At the height of demand that March and April, that would only have lasted about half a day.

Within seventeen days of the first meeting with the Chinese Ambassador, the first Aer Lingus plane carrying the treasured goods was wheels down at Dublin Airport.

'EI9019 Fáilte abhaile. Dublin ATC are proud to be guiding you home safely today. On behalf of the IAA and the entire nation I would like to express our appreciation for all you are doing during this time of need.'

'I believe they've the red carpet rolled out for you …'

Those first batches from China were instantly drawn into the spotlight. After the feeling of salvation came the reckoning. Questions immediately followed about its suitability. The HSE admitted that twenty per cent of the first consignment was not suitable for use. Another fifteen per cent was deemed usable, if not first choice for Irish healthcare staff. 'When it landed with us, rather than people breathing a sigh of relief, it moved on to news stories about it not being good enough,' says Colm Henry.

National Ambulance Service (NAS) staff, carrying out household swabbing and Covid patient transfers on top of their normal duties, were very close to the edge. Some of the supplies they received featured short arms. 'The sleeves were to here,' says one ambulance staff member in the Midlands, pointing to the middle of his forearm. 'They weren't designed for taller men or women.' Ambulances in Dublin and elsewhere were on the brink of being taken off the road due to the scarcity of protective equipment. Items of PPE were redirected, moved around defensively like pieces on a chessboard to avoid a check-mate scenario. For staff working around the clock, these small logistical changes made a world of difference to an area's ability to meet the demands of patient care and testing.

'You know the expression "Everything that can go wrong, will go wrong"? It felt like everything was going wrong. I have no idea how we got through March and April,' says one senior member of the HSE efforts.

At a Sunday press briefing in the PPE distribution centre, Paul Reid was flicking through social media as people wondered why the HSE seemed to be doing a press conference in IKEA. Standing in front of a warehouse of blue shelves and boxes, Reid, Sarah Doyle and Martin Cormican were going through the arrangements with China and demonstrating the gowns and masks that had been distributed to date.

The HSE's standard annual spend on PPE is €15 million. The deal with China Resources was €225 million. The overall spend for 2020 was in the region of €915 million. Tensions continued between the HSE, the Department of Health and the Department of Public Expenditure. By June, the HSE had spent €371m, far ahead of the €251m authorized by the Government.

Teams were working all-nighters, redeployed from the traditional circuit of HSE procurement, to work on the PPE deliveries. They'd be waiting by the phone, making sure that the teams on the ground were in position in warehouses, that what was promised was being delivered, that it made it safely onto the planes and that the planes were in the air ASAP. It was a 'frenzy'.

Throughout this time, the health service was living gloved hand to masked mouth. There were times when everything came very close to the edge. Contingency plans were drawn up on the weekend of March 11 / 12 to halve the supply of PPE to more than three thousand healthcare settings because officials were unsure about the arrival of two planes at Dublin Airport that Friday afternoon. 'It was harrowing,' says Bresnan. Those in the know were floored by the weight of what was a Dunkirk moment. The enemy was at the gate. The tools to protect our frontline weren't coming. 'After that, God knows where we'd be.' HSE teams were standing on the tarmac at Dublin Airport waiting for the cargo to land. It was that close. Everyone involved at that point speaks with clarity about the fear in the air.

The intricacies of customs and who to thank and who not to thank almost led to a minor diplomatic incident. At one press briefing from the Mater Hospital, Reid made reference to 120 million masks which had been secured from South Korea, following a phone call between Taoiseach Leo Varadkar and the South Korean President Moon Jae-in. This, he discovered, isn't how South Korea does business. Reid was the subject of urgent calls to tell him to stop publicly thanking South Korea for the masks.

The 'PPE war', as some in the health sector have described it, will be judged in the fullness of time. Sean Bresnan is adamant: 'There will come a day when we will have to give answers. The one thing I'm sure of is that every single individual involved in that response made decisions for the right reasons.'

A source close to the Health Minister of the time's view is even more blunt: 'Good luck to the PAC (Public Accounts Committee) in the future if they want to scrutinize what was brought in. It was a global pandemic, people were dying all around us. We needed PPE and the HSE got the job done.'

Privately, there was real concern in the Department of Health about infrastructure surrounding the pandemic. IT systems were a major issue – they were outdated and easily overloaded. Dr Ronan Glynn, himself a former specialist in public health medicine, puts it this way: 'There's no secret in this. We do not have the IT systems in this country. We were relying on doctors around the country who were identifying cases to report it to public health, who reported it to John Cuddihy [of the HPSC], who put it in an Excel file, and he came in and would tell us, today we have … In the early days of March, when NPHET was reporting "four women and five men with coronavirus, and they're in the east of the country", we didn't have much more information. We had no way of collecting that.'

The CIDR (Computerised Infectious Disease Reporting) case reporting system had had its day. Developed two decades ago, it was 'not capable of dealing with something as huge as this', according to Dr Tony Holohan. Worrying signals about CIDR had long been circulated to the HSE. The 2013 Report of the Pandemic Review Group into the State's response to H1N1 noted that 'there was some criticism of CIDR when difficulties arose handling large amounts of data'. There had been reviews of the software in the intervening years but the problems would once again stymie public health responses.

The delay in tackling international travel had consequences. There was no decisive early action taken on St Patrick's Day or the Cheltenham horse racing festival in the UK, where as many as 20,000 Irish racegoers were among the 250,000 in attendance. The day after the first restrictions were announced, Health Minister Simon Harris announced that people returning from Italy and Spain would be asked to restrict their movements for two weeks when they returned. The same advice would not be given to those returning from Cheltenham. One woman who contacted me at the time of the race festival told me of her husband, who spent two weeks in the spare room after he returned. She was pregnant at the time, and he had told her she was overreacting by asking him not to go. He was the only one of the group of four not to come home with coronavirus. She didn't speak to him for two weeks.

'We were allowing a frenzy to be whipped up,' says one government adviser, who argues that the decision to cancel the parades and travel to Cheltenham should have been made on the same day as the rugby match with Italy was cancelled in order to prevent unnecessary panic and confusion in the media. This, to the Chief Medical Officer's mind, was 'disproportionate' for the time. 'It didn't seem to be terribly transmissible back at that stage,' says Holohan's NPHET colleague Dr Cillian De Gascun. 'All of the imported cases seemed to be readily contained. There were no big outbreaks on aeroplanes at that stage. Even at that point you sort of thought maybe this is going to be readily sort of controllable.'

Reflecting on the earliest days of the State response, the Deputy CMO Dr Ronan Glynn says: 'There was so much we didn't understand about the virus. About how it was transmitting, particularly, and obviously we didn't know the extent to which you can transmit asymptomatically and presymptomatically [before the onset of symptoms]. That turned out to be a very significant factor.' Glynn believes if the world had been aware of how the virus transmits even a couple of weeks sooner than it was, 'it would have made a phenomenal difference. But the world didn't understand it, and it's a real shame.' Hunting only for symptoms meant that as many as half of all early cases were missed.

Ireland's response was tied in with European efforts at the time, and evidence from Europe, Tony Holohan says, was limited: 'We tried to keep an eye on what was evolving in the international evidence on travel and transmission and followed very quickly what the position of the ECDC was. From our point of view, at a European level, it was a bit more complicated; I might as well be honest. This is just a personal view – the arrival of Brexit and all of that, you no longer had the British component in the same way.'

'You didn't have the British firepower and thinking capacity in there ... I don't care what anyone else says,' says Holohan, 'Britain punched above its weight, even if it's a big country, it punched above its weight in European public health terms with the ECDC. Brexit, as far as I'm concerned, had a big effect on the European response. The solidarity of the European response was not as strong as it should have been. When you were looking for leadership and a common position at European level, it just wasn't as strong. So we were following what the advice was and the advice at the time was very much that we keep the borders open.'

Some ministers raged at the lack of direction from Europe. Simon Harris and his officials were known to be frustrated at what the EU did wrong in the early days of the pandemic. Why was there no common position on travel? Why was there nothing on testing? Why were we fighting it out for PPE?

With little clarity and unity of purpose across Europe, and with scientists here and abroad still not clear on how the virus acted or how to tackle it, the country would soon be forced to confront the reality of a twenty-first-century pandemic.

Chapter 4: A St Patrick's Day Like No Other

O'Connell Street, Dublin, 17 March 2020

Richard Quinlan was in his jeep driving down O'Connell Street, right down the centre of the traditional parade route past the GPO. Town was dead. There was no one to be seen. In any other year, even by that early hour, queues would be forming outside pubs in Temple Bar, and crowds seven or eight deep would be thronged together along the footpaths on either side of the Spire.

On St Patrick's Day 2020, the only queue or gathering of people in town was for Covid swabbing on Sir John Rogerson's Quay. The LÉ *Samuel Beckett* had been made available to the HSE two days earlier. Quinlan, the NAS's Chief Ambulance Officer for North Leinster, had arrived the day before St Patrick's Day to get them ready for what was to be something of a 'soft launch' before further rollout.

'Dock on Rogerson's Quay and await further instructions.'

The previous weeks had seen the job specification of ambulance staff turned upside down and it wouldn't be the last time. They were the first community swabbers, tasked with going to people's homes if there was a suspected case and collecting a swab to be tested.

When Richard and crew arrived in someone's driveway, kitted

54

out in PPE outside the front door, every curtain in the neighbourhood would twitch; people would peek through blinds or even come to their front doors and stare across at what was happening. Crews would park up a few minutes away from their destination and call the person to be swabbed. 'Can you isolate? Leave the front door open for us. Put your dog in another room.'

Asking people who were being tested to isolate for the coming days was often met with quizzical stares: 'What do you mean, isolate? What are you talking about?' This was all very new.

The early concerns about PPE and any lingering hesitancy about how to handle this new virus were to the forefront of crews' minds. Richard always made sure to step through the breach first – 'If the boss is doing it, well, then we all can.'

By mid-March, Quinlan's hands were raw from constant washing with hand sanitizer. You'd wash your hands three or four times for every house you swabbed in. It's a routine that will stick for many people across the country. His jeep smelled of alcohol gel. It followed him everywhere. Richard was determined not to bring the virus home to his wife and daughter. He wiped his car down several times daily.

The house call experience meant Quinlan was one of a small number of people in the country who could say they had some familiarity with dealing with the virus.

'I remember most of them were unshaven,' says Richard of the *Samuel Beckett* crew, who had just come back from sea. Throughout 2019 and 2020, they'd been performing multiple long missions in the Mediterranean, and arriving back on home soil in Dublin, only to be put on emergency duty, was a head-spinning experience. Quinlan told them the first order of business: 'Tomorrow morning, you all need to be clean-shaven to wear masks.' He remembers being met with some puzzled looks, but the crew were dedicated and ready to help.

He explained that the masks wouldn't seal properly over facial hair, and this would put not just them as individuals, but the whole ship, at risk.

Quinlan and Defence Forces personnel inspected the ship to get it ready. There was hand sanitizer everywhere. Pumps appeared all over the ship: on walls; at the bottom of the gangplank. There was a feeling of paranoia. The virus was everywhere and touching anything was a big risk, to the crew's mind. At this point in the pandemic, there was no room for risks.

Army engineers made sure there was power and light. Tents popped up on the quayside next to the vessel. Press Association pictures of the time show Quinlan directing traffic on the quays, pointing out to soldiers and sailors where to go and what to do.

Quinlan didn't have time to stop and think about the strangeness of the situation. Every day was chaotic. He'd be up at six in the morning at a city centre hotel where NAS staff were barracked in the opening weeks of the pandemic. Every day was an entirely new challenge. Eighteen-hour days, calls to coordinate the opening of a new swabbing centre, calls to coordinate home swabbing, calls about 'standard' ambulance callouts, calls to completely change their plans. The entire specification of his job was changing every day. The ambulance teams could only plan a matter of hours ahead. There was no point in thinking about tomorrow. Tomorrow would inevitably bring the unforeseen.

In the week leading up to St Patrick's Day, misinformation about the Defence Forces was rife. A viral voice note circulated on WhatsApp purporting to be from a member of the army suggested that soldiers would be patrolling the streets of Dublin from Monday, 16 March. It was swiftly debunked, but there was still an atmosphere of tension. The sight of the LÉ *Samuel Beckett* and tents being erected along the quays sparked another furious rumour spree, with all sorts of wild claims about martial law and army camps springing up in the capital.

The Defence Forces had come on board after a briefing with the HSE's Paul Reid, the Gardaí and senior government officials. Reid laid it all out on the table. The scale of the response would be immense. Field hospitals. Temporary mortuary centres. 'Any place we could get our hands on, we would turn it into a field hospital,' Reid says. The early projections told the HSE they would need somewhere in the region of 10,000 extra beds if transmission continued to skyrocket. As the meeting ended, Garda Commissioner Drew Harris approached Reid. He was going to attest all trainee Gardaí and put them on duty. Four hundred and fifty gardaí would pass out months ahead of schedule to be part of the national effort. Harris offered Reid the use of the Garda College in Templemore as a field hospital if it was required. Next to approach Reid was Vice Admiral Mark Mellett, Chief of Staff of the Defence Forces, with a similar offer. The HSE chief remembers coming away from the meeting wondering, 'Jesus, what can we use the Defence Forces for?'

Contact tracing was their first task. Pre-pandemic, Ireland's arsenal of contact tracers for communicable diseases amounted to sixty public health staff. The need now would be thousands of people. The sight of army trucks rolling up to HSE head-quarters at Dr Steevens' Hospital across from Heuston Station in Dublin prompted a few raised eyebrows and even a 'What the fuck?' of surprise from Reid as he pulled into the car park one morning.

The Defence Forces chauffeured Reid over the coming weeks. BMW loaned the HSE nine X1 jeeps free of charge during the pandemic, while Defence Forces personnel took shifts driving the HSE Chief Executive. Reid had been commuting to and from his home in County Leitrim in the early hours of the morning and late at night. After a near miss with a bollard one night on the road, he felt it was safer for someone else to take the wheel while he worked in the back.

As he stood on the deck of the *Samuel Beckett* on St Patrick's

Day, Richard Quinlan allowed himself to take it in. The long line of people awaiting their swabs shuffled forward. 'One at a time please. Keep a distance.' The twitching of blinds and the silhouettes of people in dockland apartments looking down on the battlefield below them. The photographers, perched up on high vantage points, trying to squeeze off a few snaps of people being swabbed. The silence of the city.

He was back and forth on the quay that day, making sure the Defence Forces were getting on okay and that things were churning along safely. At the early swabbings, people had a real fear, he remembers. One trick the swabbers themselves had learned was to step off to the side when they were doing the nasal swab. People had a tendency to sneeze when the swab was inserted that just-too-far-to-be-comfortable distance up the nostril. Being sneezed on by someone suspected of having Covid wasn't ideal for anyone on board.

He checked his watch at one point and had already notched 20,000 steps. His work wasn't done. Quinlan went from the LÉ *Samuel Beckett* back across the Liffey to Croke Park, where the drive-through testing had just opened. The queue of cars to the home of the GAA on the traditional day of the club championship finals was replaced by lines of vehicles containing drivers waiting to be guided through the bowels of the stadium to be swabbed.

From Croke Park he headed to Tallaght Stadium on the Southside, one of the first swabbing sites in the country. The experience of the NAS crews in Dublin was attracting attention. Calls were coming in from as far away as Donegal looking for images of how they were setting up. Services in Scotland and Wales, too, had seen the early photos of the Navy vessel in Dublin on Sky News and wanted to know how the Irish were doing it.

It was a proud day for Richard and the team. There would be harder to come.

The infrastructure around testing was already creaking. Anne O'Connor, the HSE's Chief Operations Officer, told a press briefing on St Patrick's Day that the Health Service was set to run out of swabbing equipment before a new shipment of 30,000 kits arrived on the nineteenth. Demand was far outrunning supply.

Emergency phone lines were swamped, with people concerned about their symptoms calling 999 or 112. From Friday 13 March, anyone with symptoms – regardless of their travel history – was urged to contact their GP. More than four thousand swabs were being taken every day but a maximum of two thousand test results were coming back from labs. Members of the public could wait over and beyond a week for their swab results. The HSE asked the public for patience. Capacity would soon become a flashpoint for both the Government and between NPHET and the HSE.

The streets were quiet across Ireland for St Patrick's Day, the traditional parades replaced by home efforts and virtual gatherings. Tourists wandered aimlessly around Temple Bar with only fast food outlets and shut pubs to look at.

The news of the pub lockdown had been confirmed days earlier, prompted by a furore following images on social media of revellers blaring out Neil Diamond's 'Sweet Caroline' in a Temple Bar pub. 'Reaching out … touching me … touching you …' Many publicans took the decision themselves to shutter. The Licensed Vintners Association and Vintners' Federation of Ireland were summoned to a meeting with the Health Minister on Sunday 15 March. Following the meeting, representatives of the vintners were visibly pale and shaken as they waited around the lobby trying to get the word out to their members.

It was a decision they had backed in the national interest but there was an immediate sense of what this would mean for many businesses across Ireland. Some pubs that shut their doors that Sunday would never trade again.

The idea of a St Patrick's Day speech had been germinating in the Taoiseach's mind since Washington. Details of his address were kept under wraps until just an hour before it was broadcast. Varadkar's speech was warmly received, 1,789,000 people tuning in to listen to it live on RTÉ or Virgin Media. The Taoiseach himself was taken aback by the reaction. He himself wasn't 'mad on' the speech, which, he says, was 'announcing nothing'. 'Despite what people may say about me, I am a policy wonk and a substance person.'

He came round to it somewhat when he scrolled online after the speech: 'Social media, which is generally hostile, particularly Twitter, particularly to politicians and particularly my party – just to see that suddenly turn. It was bizarre. I think Paul Donnelly, local Sinn Féin TD, kind of criticized me, exactly for the same reason I would have criticized me which is I didn't actually announce anything. He was annihilated on Twitter, and I just thought it was the weirdest thing how a medium that was so negative to us was all of a sudden defending everything I say. It was one of those moments. People call it the "Green Jersey" moment. It's wartime rather than the flag. All governments experienced that, even ones that handled the situation terribly.'

The speech was light on new measures but it was seminal and set the stage for what was to come.

'This is a St Patrick's Day like no other,' he began. 'A day none of us will ever forget. At a certain point, we will advise the elderly and people who have a long-term illness to stay at home for several weeks. We call it cocooning, and it will save many lives, particularly the lives of the most vulnerable, the most precious in our society.'

He called on families to keep their distance to protect their relatives, urging them to use Skype or FaceTime to check in with loved ones and to promise them they'd see them again soon. He thanked retail workers, hauliers who were keeping the supply lines open, the childcare staff keeping the kids of vital health workers safe, civil servants and army personnel for adapting to contact tracing.

Still on duty, Richard Quinlan listened to the speech and said the volume of ambulance callouts dropped like a stone. 'People were afraid to go to hospital. People were afraid to call an ambulance. People were afraid to go outside their door. For the first six to eight weeks, that just dropped off the scale.'

Varadkar turned the spotlight onto healthcare workers. Looking back, he said, 'I was conscious of a lot of my family working in healthcare in both Dublin and in London. London was very serious by then and I was aware of healthcare workers dying around the world. That was definitely in my mind, that we would be asking a lot of our healthcare workers including friends and family in the time ahead.'

His speech continued, 'This emergency is likely to go on well beyond March the twenty-ninth. It could go on for months into the summer so we need to be sensible in the approach we take.'

The virus was growing silently but exponentially in our communities. Whatever preparations had been made would now be put to the ultimate test.

'This is the calm before the storm, before the surge. And when it comes, and it will come, never will so many ask so much of so few.'

Chapter 5: The Mater

It was a late night under the fluorescent lights on St Cecilia's Ward in Dublin's Mater Hospital. Clinical Nursing Manager Mary Elizabeth Jones was standing at the centre of the ward with her closest colleagues and infection control experts. It was the Friday before St Patrick's Day and the hospital was taking a deep breath before the storm.

Mary Elizabeth was studying the tiniest details of how to isolate and treat incoming patients with Covid-19. How should rooms be laid out for isolating patients? What are the protocols for wearing and removing PPE? How long should it take to don and doff? Where do the bins go to prevent wider spread?

Cecilia's would be the second ward in the hospital to convert to Covid-only care. It would not be the last.

At about 1 a.m., they called it a night. Satisfied they had considered as many eventualities as they could, Mary Elizabeth and her colleagues said their goodbyes and headed for the exits. Mary jumped in a taxi underneath the entrance of the Whitty Wing on the North Circular Road, across from Mountjoy Prison. She was tired and quiet on the way home; worried about what might lay ahead. She wanted to believe it would be a 'slow burn' – patients would be admitted in ones and twos over time, the protocols would hold, there would be days before the true impact of any surge would be felt.

It wasn't to be.

The first patients in St Cecilia's Ward were admitted that very morning. On Monday, the twenty-five-bed ward was full.

* * * *

Dublin's Mater Misericordiae Hospital has seen all manner of crises since it opened in 1861, on Eccles Street in the heart of Dublin's north inner city. It is one of the longest-serving hospitals in the country, and it is woven into the fabric of the city. Almost everyone who has lived long enough in Dublin will have known someone who has worked in the hospital or who has been treated there. This connection has its advantages. 'The Mater has an institutional memory,' says Dr Gerard O'Connor, consultant in emergency medicine. 'We've been around a long, long time.'

Covid was far from the Mater's first pandemic or epidemic. In 1866, the Mater was the first hospital in the country to keep its doors open twenty-four hours a day to treat patients during the cholera epidemic. That was the first time the hospital had to deal with an influx of patients for admission. Many more disasters would follow.

Five years later, smallpox took a devastating toll. Eight hundred patients were admitted with the virus, many spreading the disease to each other while they waited for treatment in the hospital.

In 1918, the Spanish flu, the last pandemic to truly sweep across the world, hit without warning. Its first and second waves swept through Dublin and along Ireland's east coast with appalling consequences. Whole families were among the 25,000 lives lost. 'The Big Flu' took almost as many Irish lives as the First World War, and far more than the bloody War of Independence and Civil War.

There are historical rhymes in how the two pandemics have afflicted the city. The 1918 All Ireland Finals were postponed for a year due to the high risk of mass gatherings; the city's tram network ground to a halt as frontline workers went down sick. A frustrated Sir Charles Cameron, the country's leading medic of the time, begged the public to follow the guidelines, writing in the *Irish Times:* 'If the public would only wake up to the seriousness of the condition of things and avoid meeting in crowds, the risk of spreading the infection might be minimized.'

The impact of Covid on medical workers is something the 1918 pandemic foretold too. Social historian Dr Ida Milne has written about how the Mater, facing hundreds of cases every day, was forced to convert all but two wards to 'influenza only' in a battle to contain a virus that spread rapidly in cramped living conditions across the city's tenements. Hospital staff in Dublin, not least the Mater's chaplain, Fr Murray, were among the lives lost after a brutal winter surge.

So devastating was the pandemic in Dublin that Mater doctor D.W. McNamara wrote of the grim acceptance of the scale of loss in the city: 'It was a depressing job ministering to patients with such a disease, with death at every corner of every ward, and it sometimes was a negative though very real comfort to look out of one of the windows facing towards Berkeley Road of a morning and watch the cavalcade of funerals trotting quietly and inevitably towards Glasnevin. At least one felt ... bad and all as it was in the Mater ... it was just as bad everywhere else.'

Dr O'Connor says, 'We have been exposed to multiple major incidents,' pointing to the return of hospital ships with the wounded from the Great War, and combatants and civilians injured in the Easter Rising being treated for shrapnel injuries sustained in fighting and shelling across the city's Northside. These were followed in short order by the War of Independence and the Civil War, all leaving a trauma etched in the hospital's stone façade. More recently, the Dublin bombings of 1972, 1973 and 1974 and the Stardust nightclub fire on St Valentine's Day 1981 are within living memory.

O'Connor plays a lead role in both the national and hospital planning for potential events ranging from chemical or biological incidents to terrorist attacks or the arrival of dangerous contagions. His first experiences of this pandemic were in the smooth operation of training simulations. As fate would have it, in October 2019, the Mater underwent an inspection by Sir Mike Jacobs from Imperial College London, one of the western world's leading infectious disease consultants. The focus then was Ebola or any of the viral haemorrhagic fevers. O'Connor led Jacobs, alongside Mater colleague Dr Aoife Cotter, around the Emergency Department, highlighting the steps that had been taken to prevent the transmission of a very infectious virus. 'We were very fortuitous to have that work and training done early.' It was a stroke of luck that would serve them well.

When the alarm was raised about Covid in early 2020, the Mater again led the way in preparations. O'Connor ran a multi-agency dry-run simulation. They worked on what would happen if a Covid patient arrived at the hospital. For many staff, it was the first toe in the water with the many layers of heavy, burdensome PPE they would be clad in over the long months to come.

It is one thing to simulate a major incident. It is another thing entirely when it arrives on your doorstep. For senior management, there were algorithms and conversations about how bad it could get. The Mater's Chief Operating Officer, Josephine Ryan, remembers asking how many cases Ireland would see and an infectious disease consultant telling her it would be 'two, maybe three max'.

While many across the country focus on the Taoiseach's address in Washington as the moment Covid 'got real', for O'Connor and his staff there was a very different moment.

The Department of Health, in those early months, prepared guidance on when to consider a patient as potentially Covid-infected. The algorithm for hospital admissions changed on the night of 5 March. It's a detail few outside the health setting would understand the implications of. As simple as a flow chart adding a new bubble of text and a new pathway.

'This essentially said to the whole system, anywhere in Ireland, that if anyone has community-acquired pneumonia, they should be considered as Covid-19. I dragged everyone, all of my staff, into the red room. All of the Emergency Department staff, the on-calls, the doctors and nurses. They knew what this meant. It meant Covid was now spreading readily in the community. There were tears that night. People were very upset.'

On any single day, a hospital the size of the Mater could admit ten to fifteen people with pneumonia; those were the figures until that day in March. Changing the way the Irish hospital system viewed those patients – a subtle change on an A4 page – was the signal to medics that everything had changed completely. They would now need to gown up and don full PPE for each patient with suspected pneumonia.

Some people in the room cried. They knew this meant that the virus could not be controlled. It was no longer something 'over there' that could only be brought into the country by visitors or citizens returning from abroad. This was circulating in Dublin's families and offices. In cramped shared living spaces. In workplaces. In bars. In meat factories and schoolyards. This was the night that Covid-19 became different from anything they'd seen before. And it was before they had seen *anything*.

If something was spreading on the streets and in the homes of Dublin, it would not be long before the true impact was felt on the floors of the Mater. On St Cecilia's Ward, fear set in. Covid patients deteriorated quickly, far faster than the clinical teams could have anticipated. By now, we're all familiar with the notion of Covid patients gasping for air. That notion arrived very late for many people, too late for some.

Oxygen saturation, or 'sats', for healthy adults is between 94 and 100 per cent. For someone with Covid pneumonia, it can be as low as 50 per cent – half the normal figure.

Mary Elizabeth Jones vividly remembers 27 March. As families across Ireland stood outside their homes and clapped for healthcare workers, she donned PPE to enter the room of Ionuț, a Romanian man, to check his sats. There was little of obvious concern. He smiled to greet her as he continued to chat away happily to his family on the other end of the FaceTime call, reassuring them he was okay and checking in on how their day had been.

She put the sats probe on his finger. Then another. And then another.

He did not look hypoxic. 'This was a very creepy, silent thing happening to him. Most people with those levels of hypoxia would be gasping for breath.' She left the room feeling shocked. 'We need to get ICU up for review,' she told her staff nurse. Within half an hour, the man was moved to the intensive care unit.

The experience was an early example of the challenges of connecting with patients through layers of PPE. Ionuț didn't understand how dangerous his condition was. 'He tried to put on his shoes when we told him he was being moved to ICU.' He handed Mary Elizabeth the phone to explain what was happening to his son on FaceTime. 'No, sir, you have to stay where you are!' She frantically tried to shout through her mask and visor, battling to simply be understood. 'We couldn't make eye contact through double layers of visors and goggles. He couldn't understand me at all.' Ionuț would be brought to Intensive Care and intubated for ventilation. He spent the next three months in ICU.

Mary's colleague Amy got her attention, asking for another sats check on a woman in Bed 3. The woman was sitting up, eating a yogurt. She was taken to ICU in less than forty minutes. 'That night was terrifying, just terrifying,' Mary Elizabeth remembers. The nurses waited through the long night, their shifts punctuated by regular oxygen checks, afraid they might need to send another patient downstairs for intubation.

The ICU at the Mater is down on Level 3 in the same Whitty Building as Cecilia's. The building was only commissioned in 2014 – with plenty of space to keep patients apart to prevent the spread of infection. 'A godsend,' as Dr Colman O'Loughlin, ICU consultant, says. The Kerry man's earliest memories of the pandemic are Zoom calls with colleagues across Europe, particularly in Italy, warning them of what was to come. It was chilling, but Colman says that the time and the level of detail given by their Italian colleagues experiencing the full brutality of the pandemic in Lombardy was priceless.

Like his colleagues elsewhere in the hospital, Dr O'Loughlin noticed an eerie lull in early March. By now eleven years in the Mater after returning from Australia, he remembers inspecting ventilators and beds in a revamped ICU. 'We were kicking tumbleweed down the corridors,' he says. Two-thirds of the ICU was cleared to make way for the influx, ready for whatever surge came. Except there was no surge. 'We were looking at each other and blinking, really.' The scenes inside the hospital, at this point, were similar to those on the empty streets outside, as the country shut itself down to do whatever it could to protect our hospitals.

Reinforcements were making themselves available if needs be. He took a call from a retired consultant who, despite being older in years and having been warned that his advancing age would put him in the firing line of the worst impacts of the disease, said, 'There's my number, you call me when you need me.'

'These were consultants in their sixties and seventies who were saying "put me down on the roster". It was quite humbling to see that, guys seven or eight years retired putting their hands up.' Their response bolstered the feeling of 'war-time' energy in the Mater. The retired consultants here were not called into action but their offer of support bolstered those who were togged out and waiting. 'This was just one of the triggers to people that "Jeekers, we need to stand up and be counted now."'

Once it landed, there was no mistaking it.

Dr O'Loughlin says that on an average day in ICU and the high dependency unit, you could be dealing with fifteen, twenty, twenty-five different diseases across all the patients. With Covid, it was a clean sweep. Thirty-six patients with 'very, very severe lung disease'. Even at an early stage, his team were battling with a growing realization. 'It was becoming obvious to us. The ones who were getting the severe forms of this were not going to survive.' There was no cure. There still is no cure. All the teams in ICUs and wards across the Mater and around the world could offer was support. Support them with everything they could muster to prevent complications and give their immune system every chance, however slim, to beat the disease. 'All we could do is stand to the sidelines and help that immune system. But if the disease was stronger than the immune system, they wouldn't survive.'

This is what sets coronavirus apart. The immediate comparisons made with the disease are with the flu, and with pneumonia. O'Loughlin says that even with severe pneumonias, 'we tend to get people better'. With Covid, even in patients who 'should' beat it – patients in their thirties, forties and fifties – sometimes there was no telling.

'We had three people in their thirties die from this ... we get them to ICU because we think they'll survive. These cases have been very difficult. You're telling families and they're

69

saying "but this only affects old people". It doesn't. Some of these patients would have had other underlying issues or comorbidities, but not all of them. And even if they do, with those comorbidities and without Covid, you would expect them to live another thirty to fifty years. That wasn't hitting home for some people – some of these things can be even just a bit of high blood pressure, the kind of thing people live their life not realizing they have.

'What kills me is when you see these patients and they're usually in a coma so they've effectively been taken out of the equation. We have managed them medically only so much.'

These young people leave behind a void that cannot be filled. Families would seldom get the chance to say goodbye in a way they would have wanted. 'We'd have families asking if they could get their loved one to do a video call with their six-year-old. That's what kills me. It's what's left behind. These are young people who started their lives, their families and would have expected to be able to rear those kids all the way through. Through school, through college, on to get married. That's been absolutely taken away from them.'

Colman saw what it meant even in those early days of the disease. He's as experienced as they come in intensive care medicine in this country and, contrary to what some may believe, it is still hard to separate the emotions from the moment of care. He'd look at these patients and reflect on his own life, his own children. Most people he works with would do the same. 'There's families being torn apart by this disease,' he says.

The rounds continue. The scrubbing. The donning. The doffing. The caution. The footsteps. The raised voices to try to make yourself heard. On one round, he saw John, one of his patients in ICU, looking out of the window. It was a Tuesday morning. A nurse said to him: 'He's a bit upset today.'

'What's going on?'

'It's his mother-in-law's funeral.'

There was a brief second of silence that could have lasted forever. It ended in a beat: 'Tomorrow, it's his wife's funeral.'

John couldn't leave to say goodbye to the person he was meant to share the rest of his life with, or to her mother.

'He was stuck in hospital. Covid has ripped families apart.'

Colman reflects on the cruel imbalance of the disease. The fact that some people may never know they had Covid. They may never have even the slightest tickle of a cough or notice even a touch of a temperature. Others will stay at home in bed for two weeks, suffering the mild edge of this disease, perhaps losing their sense of smell and taste for a time and then moving on. For others, the disease will put them in a medically induced coma, intubated, ventilated, a machine doing all the work the machinery of their body can no longer do. For those least fortunate, it took their life or the lives of one or more of those closest to them. One woman lost her twin sister – the baby she came screaming into this world alongside – her father and her brother-in-law, all in the space of two weeks.

Many of these stories will never be told, the losses impossible to put into words. But they will stay with the staff members, never to be forgotten.

∗ ∗ ∗ ∗

PPE was a struggle in the early days of the pandemic. 'Some of the stuff we were getting at the start was less than good quality,' says Colman. 'Some of the gowns were just tearing apart. Some of the masks you couldn't breathe through … Some of the goggles would fog up, you couldn't see or they were dirty.' It was the last thing they needed. With car crashes, emergency mode can last forty minutes. For anything bigger, it can be hours. For Covid, emergency mode didn't let up for days on end.

When the PPE did arrive, it changed everything staff knew about the humanity of their jobs.

From the second you walk through the doors of the Mater Hospital in 'peacetime', the porters are among the first people you see. They walk around eight miles a day, ferrying patients on trolleys between wards, trafficking supplies and waste wherever it needs to go. Few have as many miles under their shoes as Ken A. Byrne. He has worked in the Mater for twenty-two years. 'I've to retire at sixty-five. Do you know what I'll be doing the week after I retire? Coming right back through those doors to volunteer here. That's how much I love it. I love it with a bleeding passion.' So much so, he encouraged his son Ken Jr, who's twenty-eight, to join him on the floors.

Things changed for him back in February. He noticed the fear almost immediately. Ken knows more than anyone how to read the mood of the hospital, what's on everyone's mind and how to listen to the hum of conversations. One thing he and his one hundred porter colleagues realized a long time ago was that they needed their own language. The MRSA superbug, once the biggest fear of hospital porters, became known to them as 'Mr Sa – Mister for MR, Sa for SA,' he smiles. 'You don't want patients fearing you or hearing MRSA so you use these codewords.'

What word did they use for coronavirus?

'Karachi.' Why? 'One of the lads, another porter, Paul Roche, was looking through his radio app one day and came across Karachi FM. You don't want patients hearing "Corona", they'll be panicking. I hope the city of Karachi doesn't do us for slander!'

It wasn't easy. Patients struggled to connect with porters and staff as they looked at them through masks, gowns and goggles, shouting to be heard. 'The fear of God was in us all,' says Ken. 'We got on with it.'

Byrne and his pals battled through plastics and perspex to bring the human touch back to the hospital. They stood with patients, shared jokes and stories, helped them from their chairs, allowing them to grip the porters' arms through the PPE as they stood. The sense of touch, the locking of eyes of recognition. These small things made a real difference.

* * * *

While the Mater's staff tried to make patients feel safe, they were always conscious that they themselves were not immune from the impact of the virus. When they went home, some staff slept in separate beds from their partners. Others left their families behind to protect them. Nurses were offered rooms in the Maldron Hotel. Mary Elizabeth Jones stayed there for a time, thankful to not have to stress about infecting her fiancé or her housemate. She collected her breakfast in a brown paper bag outside her room and walked out to meet whatever the day would throw at her.

Suzanne Dempsey was in the car one morning just before 7 a.m. The hospital's Director of Nursing wanted to get into work early, to make sure her charges, the hospital's 1,700 nurses, were ready and coping. She was making her way down Glasnevin Avenue, the commute to the Mater a glide through light traffic as people stayed at home.

The phone rang. 'I need to talk to you, Suzanne.' It was the Critical Care Unit's Assistant Director of Nursing. Suzanne knew from the tension in her voice that this was not good. She instinctively pulled her car over to the side of the road. 'Yep, fire ahead.'

An ICU nurse had contracted Covid and had deteriorated quickly. She had now been admitted to her own department, under the care of the people she had worked alongside for years.

73

Suzanne's heart could have stopped. 'I nearly got sick, physically sick.' She sat for the next ten minutes in her own thoughts in a state of shock. She wondered: 'Is this the start of it?' She was stunned by the reality of what Covid could do, not just to patients but to the staff too. 'This could happen to any one of us.'

All the staff in the Mater speak of how the impact of their colleagues' individual battles with Covid affected them. There are scars that do not heal.

One evening in April, around 8 p.m., Dr Colman O'Loughlin was in a meeting which included both sets of nurses – the day crew and the night team. It was a rare moment to overlap and prepare those coming on shift for the particular needs of the ICU patients of the day. The bomb dropped. One of the ICU nurses was being admitted to ICU. The nurse in question had spent over a decade working in intensive care at the Mater. Intensive care is a family. You work alongside these people in the toughest, most relentless of environments. You spend years battling alongside them, training alongside them, hearing all about their family, their kids, their husbands and wives and partners. You go for drinks with them at the end of a brutal week.

The meeting was wrenching. Tears were shed. Colman remembers that 'no matter what I said, it was going to be the wrong thing because everything was just so unsure. She was in a bed in her own ICU. All of a sudden, it was a Lombardy, Madrid or London situation.'

It drove people to the very limits of what they could do. Shifts were worked through gritted teeth and tearful eyes. It was a traumatic experience to see someone who was a constant, a role model for many younger nurses who had honed their careers in the ICU, intubated and ventilated alongside some of the sickest patients in the country. Some said they didn't want to work. They couldn't work. How could they? How could they come in to work and detach themselves from the fact that the person they were trying to pull through the dark was one of their closest comrades? But they always showed up. 'I'm not coming in tomorrow' was inevitably followed by the same nurse togging out for another day on the ward. 'They felt not just this desire to help [their colleague] but to help every other patient. They couldn't stay away. The only times they stayed away was when they were close contacts and they were told to stay away – or if they had Covid themselves. It was phenomenal.'

Mary Elizabeth Jones will never forget it: 'Will you please call my sister?' One of her closest friends and colleagues, let's call her Orla, had become sick and was urgently being moved to ICU. Mary Elizabeth couldn't believe it. Orla? Orla, who had trained her and shaped her into the nurse she was today? Mary Elizabeth was the only person on hand to help. Orla's family were halfway around the world, and her situation was rapidly taking a turn for the worse.

'I wasn't able to handle it,' says Mary Elizabeth. The ICU team made the very best efforts to reassure her: 'You've got to trust that when you go home, someone else is going to take care of her now.' She cried and cried, and she was not alone. Many people speak about nursing and healthcare being a family. Families row. Families fall out. This happens in hospitals too. There are often brusque conversations; there can be flashes of frustration. Mary Elizabeth experienced none of that this time. This was a family sick with worry about one of its own.

The ICU manager rang Mary Elizabeth that night to let her know how Orla was doing. The next morning she made sure she went down there again to see how her dear friend had been overnight. She met one of her clinical nurse specialists who had redeployed to the ICU. Mary Elizabeth needed a lot of support and she got it. It was her job to try to support Orla's family, texting and calling with updates. It was only through this that she realized that Orla's next of kin was her best friend on St Cecilia's ward.

It was a week of impossible worry. Every day, at the start of her morning update, Mary Elizabeth updated the nurses on how Orla was doing in ICU. 'You had to keep going. You had to keep going to work.'

In total, four of the Mater's nurses ended up in ICU, critically ill with Covid-19, two of them ICU nurses themselves. Both are back working in Intensive Care alongside the colleagues who cared for them in their darkest hour.

Suzanne Dempsey sums it up. 'They were ventilated for weeks up there. They were being nursed by their own colleagues. Can you imagine that? They're being cared for, turned, proned, ventilated, critically ill ... being looked after by their own colleagues.'

Orla herself returned to work three months later. 'We can't get rid of her,' says Mary Elizabeth. 'She trained me, I've looked up to her my whole career and now she's running around the place faster than me. She won't even take holidays.'

* * * *

Fear on the frontline manifests in many different ways. One of the moments Ken A. Byrne remembers most clearly is the terror he sensed from one colleague when she saw her first patient wheeled in with *Karachi*.

He wheeled a patient into a ward, the trolley squeaking on the floor. The sweat gathering on Ken's brow, his breathing heavier than normal, still adjusting to the effect of wearing a mask. Ken, the patient and the medical staff around him were all clad in PPE, 'aliens' as he puts it. Ken glanced into the kitchen as they passed. 'A pantry girl looked out, I think it was the first Covid patient they had into that ward.' The woman's face betrayed her shock. The colour drained from her face and she faltered. 'She went wax.' Ken dropped the patient into the ward, de-gowned, scrubbed up and went straight back to the kitchen. 'Are you alright, love?' No. She collapsed into a hug in floods of tears, grabbing his arms. 'My nerves are gone with this thing,' she said.

'She had young kids to be worrying about, parents to be worrying about.' He told her not to worry, that everyone was gowned up for exactly this reason. 'Do what you need to do and we'll get through it.' She eased. They went for a smoke outside. 'I'll just never forget it. The drain of colour from her face,' Ken remembers. It was the same fear that would characterize what so many felt for loved ones over the months to come.

High above Dublin, in a temporary unit attached to the roof of the McGivney Wing, is the CEO's office. From there, you can look right out across the city, across the Liffey, past the old Central Bank and St Stephen's Green, to the suburbs and the mountains; to the north, you can see Phibsboro, the crumbling grey of the Phibsboro Shopping Centre and Dalymount Park, out as far as the airport. If the senior management of the Mater ever lost sight of just how many potential patients were out there to be looked after by their staff, a few minutes of quiet reflection looking through the glass would remind them.

In the CEO's office, there is a whiteboard. It's more of a wall than a board, growing over time with the addition of new resources and complexities to be worried over. It filled up with lists – of bed numbers, of wards, of sheer numbers. CEO Alan Sharp and COO Josephine Ryan looked at it every hour, every day, trying to picture what was needed and where they could divert resources to those in most need. Alan initially felt that Covid would be a slow roll. Pausing for a moment, he smiles wryly: 'No chance of that.'

The National Isolation Unit was the first port of call on his board. It was soon full. Next it was St Agnes's Ward, then St Cecilia's ... and then more. On early Zoom calls with the hospital management and senior clinical team, concern was palpable. Heated discussions were had about whether there was enough. Enough oxygen to keep ventilated patients alive. Enough PPE to keep staff safe and well. Enough beds to keep patients in a comfortable and isolated setting.

Amid a national surge in demand for PPE, and with the HSE scrambling to find new supply chains in China and South Korea, the situation became stark: 'We came within one day – one day – of running out of facemasks.' The hospital's charitable arm went to work seeking donations; procurement teams worked around the clock trying to find leads on gowns and gloves from businesses in Dublin, or anywhere around the world for that matter. The hospital's head of procurement, Seamus Priest, was constantly on the phone, at one point teaming up with a local sewing factory that would modify unsuitable PPE as it arrived, just to try to make sure that anything that could be used would be used.

'It was a period of great concern,' says Alan. Staff were falling sick. More still were being ruled out of work as close contacts. If there are no staff, the outcomes for patients are a lot tougher to manage. On one single day, 450 staff members were ruled out of action. Alan and Josephine often took whatever opportunity they could to move around the hospital safely to ascertain what was needed and to see how the exhausted staff were coping in the heat of a pandemic none of them ever expected to face. The weight of the decisions that had to be made were enormous.

The deaths from Covid started to rise, and rise quickly. Extra cooler units were ordered in to store bodies. 'When you have to start doing that, you know you're in trouble.' With patients dying and staff falling ill, Alan signed off on the authorization. The dark thought crossed his mind, 'The next one could be for me.'

Health workers were run off their feet. Their neck-worn

bleepers buzzed constantly with calls for emergency assistance at all hours of the day. The first wave was 'hell', says Suzanne Dempsey. 'The wards had a lot of elderly patients, who sadly did not make it.' Visitor restrictions and infection control meant visiting was limited to the most extreme, palliative moments. Patients deteriorated quickly. Often in a matter of three or four hours. 'By the time you're making phone calls, it's too late.' Some older people died alone, with only the nursing staff alongside them, watching over them, praying for them in their final moments.

The devastation is impossible to comprehend. Dempsey remembers one conversation with a clinical nursing specialist on a Covid ward one Sunday. 'There were four rooms in a row and they are all relations. Husband. Wife. Sister. Brother. They nearly lost a whole family.' It is difficult to contemplate. 'The girl was due to get married herself. You're going through the contrast of planning a life and then a whole family wiped out.'

Staff of all grades were in the line of danger from Covid-19. HSE statistics show that nurses and healthcare assistants (HCAs) were at most risk. Patricia Prades, a HCA originally from the Philippines, has been in the Mater for over twelve years, having previously worked in nursing homes. The opportunity to move to an acute hospital, with better salary and benefits, is what attracted her to the job. She was not placed in direct contact with suspected Covid patients. In those earliest days of the pandemic, with PPE at a premium and understanding of transmissibility limited at best, staff away from the coronavirus pathway were wearing standard equipment. If patients didn't show symptoms of Covid, they weren't getting swabbed.

Patricia was working on Our Lady's Ward, feeding an older man who had limited vision. She remembers sitting with him and chatting to him for fifteen or twenty minutes. He was eating slowly. It was pleasant, chatting to him about his life and about what was happening elsewhere in the hospital with Covid.

A few days later, she started to feel dizzy, like she had a headache she couldn't shake. Her manager asked if she was feeling alright and sent her home when she realized she was feeling unsteady. Luckily, Patricia's home is well kitted out for self-isolation. When she got home from work, she had her husband get the log cabin they had in the back garden ready for her. Initially, she was in denial. 'I can't have Covid.' It was a strange experience at first, her husband having food delivered to her outside the log house in the garden. 'It was like being a dog, leaving the food outside!'

After a week she deteriorated and felt as if she was going to die. She panicked about her kids (aged twenty-seven, seventeen and twelve) – would she be leaving them? 'I had one foot underground already.' It was the hardest moment of her life, she says. She phoned her two youngest kids, who were in the house, looking in at them through the back window, waving at them and making sure they had eaten their dinner. It was a frightening experience. Her husband was self-isolating inside, in his bedroom, having himself become infected through Patricia.

At times she felt her chest was about to cave in. The weight of breathing was too much for her. She was terrified. Even getting to her feet was an individual battle to be overcome every few hours as she reached for water and paracetamol. 'I couldn't do it. I was shivering, I had a high temperature. I felt so weak.' She would spend the next two weeks in her log cabin. Every day looking through the back window and into the house to her kids. Finding more and more strength in her body until she was clear and ready to return to the front. There, her colleagues were battling through exhaustion to keep the hospital running.

* * * *

Heather Hawthorne is a social worker at the Mater. The role of social workers at the hospital took on an added importance during Covid, helping to keep patients in touch with their loved ones even in their darkest hours of isolation. It was not always possible, but whenever it was, the social workers made sure that compassionate visits were allowed even when the hospital itself was effectively cut off from the wider world. 'I remember it was almost like a fortress,' she says. 'Security was on the door. You had to show your pass. Everyone was wearing masks, the corridors were just completely silent.'

Because nurses were relentlessly in and out of PPE, moving between patients in isolation, the social workers took on the role of communicating between patients, the staff and the families on the outside. Families would naturally be sick with worry. 'Has my dad eaten?' 'Did he get dressed?' 'Was mam able to get out of bed?'

Calling the same family members at least once a day for many weeks, Heather remembers building up personal connections, drawing quite close to them. This meant the sometimes inevitable calls with bad news were unimaginably tough. 'Whenever you had phoned somebody every day, and you thought maybe that patient was getting better, and then unfortunately, as is the nature of Covid, sometimes people didn't and sometimes things changed very quickly – that was tough. That was really, really tough.' One patient, Sean, was admitted initially after contracting Covid in another setting. 'Every day I'd be phoning his daughter and then, unfortunately, he deteriorated quite a lot. At that time, there was a lot of talk of when the family member could come in.'

One of the first times it really hit Heather was when that woman was told she could come in to say goodbye. Heather was quickly up and down in lifts and on escalators between wards and the hospital door whenever people were allowed in for palliative visits. She'll never forget standing with that

81

daughter as she was talked through the gowning process for PPE. 'The nurse was just so lovely. She was sitting her down and saying, "You have to do this, you can't touch this. You can only stay for 15 minutes." It was so clinical.'

For someone working with people, trying to bring them closer together, the PPE was a barrier that brought home just how strange and desperate the situation was becoming. 'You had this woman, this daughter, all she really wanted to do was to come in and touch and hold her father' in his final days. The next day the phone rang. It was Sean's daughter. She was 'phenomenally thankful' to be able to get in and see her dad for even the shortest time before he died.

In those sombre moments, Heather and the social workers went to huge lengths to bring connections to those who were isolated. FaceTime and other video calls were facilitated, older patients' faces lighting up at the sight of grandchildren yelling 'Hi, Granny!', a cry that usually would have been met with the warmest of hugs. Any way that could possibly be found to bring patients and their families together was sought out. Infection control protocols meant most care packages were a no-go. Cards and hard copies of photographs were a challenge in a Covid environment. Social workers, whenever it was possible, would print out email messages or copies of photos sent from worried families, trying to bring a little colour, a little piece of home into the most sterile environment.

There were heart-warming moments in all the suffering. One man, who was admitted from a local nursing home, got a letter from his wife every single day without fail. His wife had visited him every day when he was in the nursing home, something that was ruled out by Covid visitor restrictions. Now, in the Mater, there was an opportunity to try to bring them closer together. The patient could no longer read. His vision had deteriorated over the years. Every day his wife would write the letter and one of the HCAs would go in and read it to him. It was a beautiful thing, a real lift for everyone who had the opportunity to witness it. The knowledge that there was a letter there, the privilege of the HCA to get to go in and read it. As a morale boost, it was unmatched. Happy tears were few and far between in those days. Moments of kindness made all the difference to those for whom no end was in sight.

The Mater's first wave continued right through April, tailing off in May. The hospital had seen the worst, and delivered its best in return. Reflecting on the toll it took on all of them is a heavy task.

Among the toughest moments for porter Ken were the silent journeys to the mortuary, with only the beeping of the lifts or the shimmer of distant conversations for company. 'It was hard,' he says. Ken, one of the most animated talkers you could imagine, slows to a crawl. He pauses, puffing out his cheeks and raising his hands to the back of his head, the emotional return to March and April weighing heavily on him.

'You just had to get used to Covid. It was everywhere. It was every second person. Many, many, many times I'd have gone to the mortuary. It's just a sad part of life in the hospital. But when you're putting the body down with all this gear on you; when you're looking at a patient that's dead with Covid, it was … it was a different feeling. It's never normal.' Ken falls silent. 'You felt afraid, I suppose,' he says. 'Still afraid.'

He says he felt sorry for those patients and was absolutely adamant in the line of his work that he would treat them with the utmost respect and decorum. He would bless every one of them individually. He just wanted to make sure they were looked after.

How does he feel looking back on those days? 'Horrible,' he says, his eyes glassing over. 'Horrible. Fucked.'

* * * *

On 21 April, as the pressures continued to mount on the teams working at the Mater, another doctor arrived for his shift in the Emergency Department, closing the door of his car behind him. His name was Dr Syed Waqqar Ali.

Chapter 6: Dr Ali

The Mater Hospital, Dublin, 21 April 2020

Dr Ali parked his car and kept his ticket with him, locking the door as he set off across the car park to the Emergency Department. The doting father had been planning a surprise for little Zahra, eight, the youngest of the five children he had raised with his wife Rubab. He had been eyeing up the Easter eggs in the shops, trying to decide which one she'd most like. Zahra had been waiting patiently for her dad to come home and help her finish the puzzle they'd started together before he went to work on the Covid frontline. Dr Ali said his hellos to everyone as he walked across the car park. A friendly and approachable guy, he was a kind and courteous doctor and colleague who was well liked by everyone who'd come across him over many years working as a medic in Ireland.

The Ali family, from west Dublin, were so proud of their father's efforts working with patients with Covid, but they weren't without worry. Sammar, his eldest daughter, was going through her final exams in medical school as the pandemic set in. She'd tell him she was really worried that something would happen to him. 'No, Sammar, this is what being a doctor is about. You have to be there for your patients.'

He sent her photos of himself clad in his new PPE from

outside the Mater's Emergency Department. Sammar felt her heart swell as she proudly passed her phone to show her friends her frontline hero. Her dad had always been a mentor, warmly encouraging her and helping her when she had questions about navigating med school life, working with her through topics she hadn't yet grasped, soothing her when she suffered panic attacks around exams. Sammar had always looked up to her dad, her idol, and together they were planning her first steps for after graduation that summer. They wanted to work together. Her first steps as a doctor would be alongside the person who had inspired her from a young age and constantly reminded her, no matter how difficult things were: 'Sammar, you can do it.'

The real reason Dr Ali had taken the photos of his PPE was to reassure his wife that he was okay. He worried about Rubab too. She was medically high-risk and he had been keeping a distance from the kids, always reminding them of the importance of being safe and protecting their mum.

That day, 21 April 2020, as Dr Ali arrived for work, something wasn't right. The two nurses he met looked back at him and panicked. He looked unwell, and he was beginning to feel it, too. He sat down and they swabbed him for Covid.

Sammar's phone rang. She answered and was shocked to hear her mum, crying. The Mater had called asking for Dr Ali's blood group, any allergies he might have. It was all happening so fast. Communication was hard. He'd left his phone at home that day. Sammar called the hospital to find out what was going on. The next day, Dr Syed Waqqar Ali tested positive. Once he was able to contact his family, he reassured them. He'd treated patients with Covid and wanted his family to know he'd be safe.

The family video chatted often after he was admitted as a patient. Sammar cried when she saw her father, who was never one to complain, struggling to breathe. On the video calls, Zahra would say 'I need you to smile for me, Dad.' The

Alis kept a screenshot of Dr Ali beaming from his bed for his littlest daughter, still putting his kids first.

That night, Sammar and her brothers figured out how to screen-record video chats on iPhone and were planning to do it the next time their dad could FaceTime them. A memento of the time their doctor became a patient. They never got the chance. Dr Ali had been transferred to ICU and put on a ventilator. It was a shock they had not expected and extremely upsetting. Sammar contacted people who had been ventilated before; she called the hospital multiple times a day, asking all sorts of questions about what his oxygen requirements were. The Alis prayed and prayed and prayed.

At home, Zahra was cut off and confused. Her mum had now tested positive. So had her brother. They were both isolating in their own rooms. Resting her head on her mother's bedroom door, she'd call through: 'Mum, when can I hug you again?' She had no idea what was going on. Her dad was in hospital, and not around to take her on their day trips. Zahra would plan shopping trips for the pair of them. He couldn't just go down to Lidl in his joggers – she'd plan out his outfit and get him to go down with her in his suit and tie to get her a Kinder egg. Now, though, everything was different. Everyone at home was wearing masks and gloves. Both her parents were sick, her brother was sick and her big sister was busy finishing her final exams.

Sammar kept calling the Mater. 'The minute I hung up and asked how he was, I just waited until I could call again and see how he was.' Things were deteriorating. Any time there was a glimmer of hope that he might come off the ventilator, he'd worsen again. It became a summer of panic and hurt for the Alis. Sammar had taken on responsibility with the hospital to consent to things like a tracheostomy. Once they were allowed to visit, they'd pass their dad's car in the car park every time. Sammar would look at it and think to herself: 'He's going to drive home, nobody else is going to touch it, he's going to validate his ticket and leave. We aren't going to touch it until he's coming home with us.'

When Sammar got her diploma, she spoke down the phone to the person she wanted to share it with most of all in the world. She cried down the line to her father in the Mater ICU. What should have been one of the happiest moments of her life was now one of the cruellest. But from the moment they were born, Dr Ali had told his children that, no matter what happened in life, they should never give up. He made sure his children always stayed positive in the face of life's troubles. He was fighting hard, he was still there, and she would fight on for him.

In June, Dr Ali had asked for his German CD, which was in his car. He was a polyglot and fascinated by languages, always looking for the next one to learn. Sammar had been learning German with him before he was admitted to hospital. When the family went out to get it for him, they couldn't believe their eyes. In the back seat, piled high, was a stack of Easter eggs for Zahra. He had planned to surprise his daughter with them after his shift finished back in April. It was surreal. Sammar's mind was racing to try to process everything that had happened since: 'He drove here, he parked, he walked through the car park on his own two feet, he kept his parking ticket and was going to pay it when he got out … That just, that just never happened. He never got to. When he put his feet up on the bed on April the twenty-first, he never got to take them down.'

Dr Syed Waqqar Ali's sixtieth birthday was just around the corner. The Alis had been looking forward to this milestone for quite some time and had planned to go all-out. This wasn't what they'd planned. At home they'd gone out and bought supplies to make him the biggest card they could – A1 paper, colours, glitter, everything. It was a nice distraction for the youngest and a time when they could do something hopeful together once more.

Arriving at the hospital, excited by the idea of how happy Dr Ali would be to see their card in just a few days, they were brought back down to earth with the most devastating news. On 20 July, the staff told the family Dr Ali wasn't getting better and it was time to switch to palliative care. Sammar looked at her father's face, his vitals on the monitor. She felt physical pain. Her heart was breaking. The family stayed with him. Whenever he opened his eyes, one of them would be right beside him holding his hand.

They spent those long hours talking to him. Thinking back to all the precious memories they had of him. The trips he took with Rubab when they were first married. What it must have been like for him, as the obstetrician on call, to actually deliver Sammar and her eldest brother. Who was the most troublesome as a child. Dr Ali smiled for them. Through it all, he still smiled.

When the decision was made to turn off the machine, Sammar rested her head on the pillow beside her dad's, just as she always did at home. She used to rest her head on his shoulder and ask him for advice on medical questions, or when he'd proudly show off the new stamps he'd ordered online for his collection. 'Don't tell your mum,' he'd smile.

Dr Syed Waqqar Ali died on 21 July, after three months in ICU, two days before he would have turned sixty. 'I didn't expect to be getting him flowers in this way on his sixtieth birthday,' says Sammar.

Immediately, messages of support and sympathy began to roll in. In the Mater's Emergency Department, Dr Ger O'Connor captured a moment of silence from all staff – heads bowed, their goggles and masks facing the ground – as they turned over from night shift to day, sharing the photo on Twitter. It remains difficult to talk about. 'It was our darkest day,' he says. 'For the whole country, it was a dark day.'

Online, the tributes mounted. Sammar scrolled through

them hour after hour. They were from colleagues, remembering his diligence and kindness in Navan Hospital; from the families of past patients: 'Denise, this is the lovely doctor who was there when your daddy was in hospital when Penny was only tiny. He was a gentleman. He asked to hold her and she was full of smiles for him. He remembered her when he met her again some months later.' Others shared memories of him apologizing to them for overhearing him on the phone fighting for the best treatment for them. Another read: 'He saved my son's life nine years ago, he was an amazing doctor and I will forever be grateful to him.' One woman living with a disability said that she had never felt so seen or heard by a doctor before she met Dr Syed Waqqar Ali. She wrote about how when she used to go to the hospital, doctors would ignore her and look to her sister to speak for her. Dr Ali, she said, was the first doctor to look directly at her when he was speaking, letting her know that she was the focus of his attention, and this meant so much to her.

Dr Ali always went the extra mile, staying hours longer than he needed to, often to the consternation of his family. Deep down, however, they loved his dedication. His commitment to seeing his job through and protecting his patients.

In Islam, it is customary for bodies to be buried as early as possible. Sammar remembers asking if it was possible to bury him immediately or to wait until the twenty-fourth, adamant that he shouldn't be buried on his birthday. In the end, they just didn't have a choice. He was buried on the day he would have turned sixty. Little Zahra didn't really know what was going on until the day of the funeral. Then she cried and cried. Sammar's focus that day was on minding Zahra and her mother. It was a devastating day.

Many remember the statement Sammar gave on RTÉ News the day her father died. Outside the family home, Sammar stood with her family behind her, united as they always have been and always will be, Zahra standing alongside her big sister before retreating back into her brothers' arms. 'People are only finding out now that he's a hero,' Sammar said, 'but he's been a hero to us our whole lives.'

In these moments, Sammar might have let her memory flash back to everything her father taught her. The moments her dad knew she would be a doctor when, at the age of three or four, in Pakistan, she would accompany him on calls or at clinics. Even at that age, she was taking it all in. She heard all the questions Dr Ali would ask his patients: 'How are you doing? What symptoms have you had?' One question he asked was 'Are you urinating okay?' As a knee-high child, Sammar would walk around asking people if they were urinating okay and what colour their urine was. It was one of her dad's favourite stories to tell people throughout his career and her studies. It would be a great story for him to tell patients and staff when they finally, after all those years, got the chance to work together. That dream, their dream, was taken away by Covid.

Standing outside the family home, she paused and thought about what her father would want her to do. He'd want her to be a doctor. 'Don't wait until it happens to you to realize how severe it can get,' she told anyone watching. 'Our father went to help people – he lost his life helping people – but don't take risks, don't take chances, life is too precious. There is still a Doctor Ali and she will carry on his legacy.'

Chapter 7: The Wave Breaks

While one of the central narratives throughout the Covid crisis has been that of 'Government versus NPHET', there is another battle that has been waged under the radar. It's characterized by blow-ups in meetings, briefing and counter-briefing and a tug of war over who is responsible for what and who sets the yardstick of success. It's a shadow conflict between the top table of the Department of Health's Covid response and the HSE.

Tensions between the HSE and the Department are long-standing. There have been many occasions during this pandemic when, despite their shared objectives, the organizations and the individuals who work for them have clashed. Dr Tony Holohan and Paul Reid are not close collaborators. Their relationship is 'very difficult', says one person on the Department side. The CMO of the Department of Health and the HSE's CEO have grappled on many occasions, often through proxies, about the direction of Ireland's response to the biggest health crisis of a generation and about who was ultimately responsible for setting the path out of the mire.

The testing debacle was the first time this clash of personalities rose above the surface. Ireland and other countries scrambled for the vital components of lab testing, with the HSE unable to cope, the inability to meet demand leading to backlogs and confusion over the scale of transmission and how to direct resources to meet it. The CMO, Tony Holohan, set a target at a NPHET meeting for 100,000 tests to be completed per week. It was a goal Holohan then announced at the evening press conference. HSE CEO Paul Reid was watching proceedings and was far from pleased. The feeling, shared by others alongside him in HSE management, was that Holohan was stepping far beyond his boundaries in publicly setting a target for the health service without previous agreement.

Reid would describe his own temperament as 'fiery' when needed, and on this occasion, according to many accounts, he went ballistic. The HSE's Chief Clinical Officer, Dr Colm Henry, was sitting up the table from Holohan at the press briefing when the screen of his phone on the desk in front of him lit up. It was a text from Reid. Henry's boss was infuriated by the commitment given by Holohan, reprinted in the accompanying press release and restated at the briefing that evening, Friday 17 April. He had not been consulted. Members of the HSE Executive Management team say Reid went 'berserk' and there were 'massive conniptions behind the scenes'.

'They're two very different people. Two very different styles.'

'If only the HSE was able to do this, then we'd be able to do that. It's a culture of blame.'

A source close to Reid says it was a 'tough weekend. (A) It was announced at a press conference and (B) [Paul] got on and said "what the f***? That wasn't what we agreed yesterday morning at a meeting with Martin Fraser."'

Ciarán Devane, the Chairperson of the HSE, is described by many as a very mild-mannered and courteous person to deal with. His letter to Minister Simon Harris was 'as close to a stinker of a letter as Ciarán could write on behalf of Paul'. In it, he expressed concern that 'operational requirements have at times not adequately been considered at the centre of NPHET's decision making'. Typically of Devane, he finished by lavishing praise on the Minister, the CMO, the Secretary General and the Department as a whole, 'hugely admiring' the leadership they had shown, but adding, 'with some thoughtful improvements to engagement that hard work will only be more impactful'.

Reid's letter, to the Secretary General of the Department, was less verbose and a lot less flattering. He was 'extremely disappointed' by Holohan's actions. 'Regrettably, I was taken very much by surprise' by the NPHET press briefing and the letter from Holohan that followed it. He said the directions were 'at odds' with the process agreed at the Cabinet Committee and the HSE Board's process.

A 'Come to Jesus' meeting was organized by Minister Simon Harris, who was effectively landed with the role of referee between Holohan and Reid. 'I was in the middle of it,' says Harris, 'it was inevitable.'

The meeting was blunt in the extreme. Reid let loose about being held responsible for targets that he says he told Holohan couldn't be met, and that he was being set up. 'We decided what's done is done. They virtually kissed and made up and it was fine. I think Paul had every right to blow a gasket on that, probably on balance, but look, they got on with it.'

In mid-April, when the letters row broke out, Holohan was operating on speed. Those with knowledge of his thinking at the time felt he was of the view that the HSE's senior management was not preparing for the crisis in the correct way. 'The HSE doesn't understand this disease,' was the damning verdict of one of the CMO's confidantes. 'You don't respond to a public health crisis by building graves. You may need them. But the focus needs to be on prevention.'

There is a view among some high-ranking officials in the Department of Health that at the beginning of the pandemic the HSE should have been looking at testing capacity; strengthening local contact tracing and the case reporting system; and resourcing public health teams (themselves in a long-standing industrial relations row) to take a much more visible role, and allowing them to take meaningful decisions. 'This did not happen.' Instead, it was all about 'ICU capacity, army uniforms, mortuaries, and all that shite.'

'It's a question of understanding,' says one HSE member. 'Personality clashes are one thing but it's a question of understanding. It's important that Paul has an understanding of this. He has a better understanding of it than he did but he doesn't have a background in healthcare from public health.'

'There's a lot of animosity there,' says one HSE team member close to Reid. 'They resurface today again [in the summer of 2021] and it's tiring, it's a distracting business.'

One person with knowledge of the back and forth said that at crunch NPHET meetings, the HSE delegates could go in and 'get the shit kicked out of them by Tony' and then leave the meeting to go and 'get the shit kicked out of them by Paul' for not standing up to Holohan.

Tensions between agencies and their departments, particularly in crises, can always spill over. This was, however, according to a number of different sources, deeply distracting and a different order of tension entirely.

Senior political figures were all too aware of the differences, even at an early stage of the pandemic. One minister described Holohan and Reid as 'two alpha males, marking their respective patches'. The minister ultimately responsible for handling both of them at the time of the testing row, Simon Harris, was under pressure to keep both happy. 'I was just adopting the approach of "I don't really care. Can you just get this done?"'

The debates at the time between the CEO of the HSE and the Secretary General of the Department of Health, Jim Breslin, went along the lines of Reid telling Breslin that NPHET should have a view and give a view, but NPHET should not cross the line of telling the HSE how to do things.

There has been disquiet in the Department about the rows with the HSE. One senior member within the fold said that, even stepping back from NPHET and Holohan, 'the Department of Health's role needs to be redefined. Are we there to hold the HSE accountable? Or there to watch what the HSE is doing? The lines of accountability have gotten very blurred. Someone needs to redefine the relationship in the years to come.'

Professor Philip Nolan, NPHET's head of modelling, says that there will always be a 'challenging relationship' between a government department and an agency that reports to it. 'There are enormous tensions there. We did frequently see tensions between a policy need as NPHET saw it and as the Department of Health saw it, and operational challenges ... and given the speed at which things had to move, you can easily imagine how the HSE would perceive it as unhelpful to be issued with an instruction on a Friday night.' Most of the time, he said, the tensions were worked out collaboratively rather than 'erupting' into anything, with the relationship between Holohan and Dr Colm Henry cited as a strong point, despite the 'extraordinarily difficult situation'.

One NPHET member said: 'God help us. I won't speak for anybody else. Personally, I find that man [Reid] very challenging. I think that was just a common experience. I can't put my finger on what it is exactly but I think probably he doesn't like being told what to do.'

One element of mistrust between senior HSE and NPHET originated from the make-up of NPHET. Some members of the HSE were upset, suspecting Holohan of hand-picking the membership of the group while leaving out pertinent viewpoints. The omission of Professor Martin Cormican, the national clinical lead on infection control, is seen by many as a bad mistake NPHET made in its early days. 'It was a glaring, glaring gap and many people commented on it,' says one long-standing NPHET member. 'He's a straight talker and a really clear thinker. He isn't a political creature. He'll be honest and he would call Tony out quickly on stuff he doesn't agree with. He wasn't appointed to NPHET.'

Professor Cormican himself says he wouldn't want to focus on his personal feelings, but noted that he believes the 'lead for Infection Prevention and Control, whether it's me or anyone else, is fundamental to managing a pandemic of an infectious disease. I don't understand that. I have never understood why the HSE Clinical Lead for IPC wasn't involved from the outset. It was a source of considerable disappointment to our whole team, about our discipline and what we were doing. Infection prevention and control needed to be at the heart of this. We got our heads together early on and said "We're not the ones who are important here and we're going to do our job." We wrote the guidance. It was often presented to NPHET by people other than the people who wrote it. That was disappointing. That was not something we could control and it wasn't going to get in the way of us doing our best.'

Holohan, at multiple NPHET meetings, called out the HSE for, in his view, not creating a responsive regional public health system. According to sources, he would take his glasses off and ask questions to which he already knew the answer. 'What has the HSE done about lab capacity since our last meeting? When will the HSE do something about local responses?' It was awkward. Heads would drop and officials would often look away to avoid eye contact.

The HSE weren't the only ones to have issues with Tony Holohan. Internally, in the Department of Health and even on NPHET, many officials were nettled by his methods. The CMO divided loyalties. To some he could almost do no wrong. He was kind and asked about their families; a workaholic who was in early and whose office light was still on at nine or ten o'clock at night. He had two private secretaries; notably, the minister and secretary general only have one. In the early months of the pandemic, he'd arrive into the office in running gear, his breakfast ready for him at his desk, often two boiled eggs, coffee and orange juice.

To detractors, he was 'authoritarian'. There were whisperings on corridors of tempers lost in the heat of the pandemic, of occasional blowouts of frustration, with the HSE often the target.

'He showed people a lack of respect,' says one senior NPHET member, 'particularly the HSE. There'd be torturous long meetings with a predetermined outcome. I didn't warm to him. We have to work together.'

'I like Tony and I've always worked well with him,' says another, 'but we've never needed to clash. If you are not doing what he wants in his way, he will clash and you will not come out the better for it.'

The picture painted of Holohan by critics in the health sector is of a man who could show temper and who may not have had the most constructive of relationships with people he didn't feel were useful to him. 'He might think a person is no value in a meeting,' says one senior figure, 'or have no respect for that person's opinion. And it becomes very clear.'

The criticism is tempered somewhat by many of those same people. 'Back in March and April, though, that was probably needed. He had a clear sense of direction and knew what was necessary to do. He never compromised. There's a downside to that, clearly, but he never compromised from what he felt was the right thing to do.'

Speaking of NPHET press briefings, the source says: 'There'd be days where I'd think, "We're really fucked now over X, Y or Z" and he'd have absolutely no fear about those situations. He shows astonishing courage. Fear is alien to him. I have never seen him afraid, even on the worst days. You can draw courage from people like that. When you're going to war you need a general and you need to know who's in charge. The only person we had in the arsenal who had that personality was

Tony Holohan. I genuinely don't think we'd have got through it without him.'

* * * *

As Ireland was hammered by the initial stages of the pandemic, the school closures and early restrictions of 12 March would not be enough.

The first full 'stay at home' lockdown was announced on Friday, 27 March by the Taoiseach, Leo Varadkar. Over 2,100 cases had been confirmed and there had been at least twenty-two deaths. Admissions to intensive care had doubled. Community transmission was now accounting for more than half of all cases. Clusters of infection were on the rise, with the Taoiseach making reference for the first time in a major address to nursing homes and residential care settings.

The situation was bleak. Gatherings of any number of people outside a single household were prohibited. Non-essential businesses were shut. Cocooning was introduced for those over the age of seventy. A rigid two-kilometre travel limit was brought in for all but essential purposes.

There was no question in anyone's mind that this was necessary. There are fine margins in the handling of pandemics when lives are at risk and the slightest delays can prove fatal. That evening, as Holohan stood shivering in the cold courtyard of Government Buildings awaiting an interview with RTÉ News, he was preoccupied by the number of people admitted to intensive care units. 'It peaked out at over a hundred and fifty. If we had waited another day or two [to increase restrictions], or if we had waited until the following Monday and some people were saying "Why did you come back on the Friday? Why not wait until Monday?" I think we would have breached our ICU capacity. We would have breached it.'

Professor Philip Nolan agrees. 'We came that close,' he says, pinching his fingers for emphasis, 'to having what they had in Italy. A couple of days, maybe a week of delay and we would have been overwhelmed. We would have had a thousand people requiring ICU and only been able to look after five hundred of them.' He says that, to some degree, chance saved Ireland from the fate of northern Italy. 'Chance has been really important throughout the pandemic. These things are like throwing a match into a fireworks factory. It'll either take or it won't. It literally is just random. It's a question of chance as to whether Person A decides to go to their singing practice or go to the pub or whatever it might be. There's a huge amount of randomness.'

The NPHET meetings were strained. Professor Nolan, leading the modelling, was staggered by the potential disaster that was unfolding before his eyes. 'The number of times that I have looked at a number and then had to go back and check it, because at face value the number is unbelievable. That was a weekly occurrence ... We were trying to glean information from what was going on in Italy and in China. People look back at the early models of tens of thousands of deaths and tens of thousands of cases per day and ridicule them. That was the "do-nothing" scenario. It's only the extraordinary things that have happened over the last year that have kept that, to a certain extent, at bay. I'll never forget watching the number of people in intensive care and just going "No" to myself. It literally went from thirty to seventy to a hundred and fifty in steps of three to four days. It was stuck at a hundred and fifty and we were wondering if it was stabilizing or if it was the point before it gets infinitely worse. That was the most hair-raising moment.'

In the minister's office, a depressing routine was becoming established. Simon Harris had come to dread the window between four and six p.m.. At any moment during that time on any given day, Tony Holohan would knock on the door carrying the latest update on paper or on his phone ahead of its release to the public. It made the rising cases, and deaths, all too real.

In the Taoiseach's office, Varadkar also felt that things were approaching the point of no return. He had considered invoking a constitutional state of emergency, but the attorney general informed him that there was no provision for such a move outside of a time of war or armed rebellion. He feared the measures in place wouldn't be enough to stem the tide of loss. 'There was a period where we'd introduced the restrictions but it wasn't getting any better. The number of cases, the number of deaths were still rising.' It was exponential growth in wicked efficiency. Three cases become nine cases. Nine cases become eighty-one cases. Eighty-one become 6,561. The Taoiseach was at the mercy of the spike. 'None of us knew how bad it was going to get.'

On an April visit to Citywest Hotel, which had been leased by the HSE, Varadkar and Harris were walked through what would soon become a field hospital for Covid patients. In the echoing chasm of the conference hall, they thought back to the election counts and Ard Fheis speeches given to thunderous applause from delegates in that same hall. It would now be associated with a very different emotion. 'Holy shit,' Harris thought, scanning the room imagining cot beds of sick people and mask-clad medics darting about trying to save lives. HSE officials, being shown around the site for the first time, were hit by the gravity of the situation. 'Out here, we have the mortuary,' one staff member was told. She burst into tears. Officialdom was staring a colossal human catastrophe in the eyes.

Meanwhile, in some GP surgeries, the situation was becoming strained. In Ashbourne, County Meath, Dr Maitiu Ó Faoláin got a text on a Sunday evening from a GP colleague who was in the know telling him to run down to Woodies and get a facemask – stocks of PPE were declining. Ó Faoláin scurried down the road at 5.30 p.m., racing to get to the hardware store

101

before it closed at six. He grabbed hold of six pairs of goggles and the two remaining gardening facemasks.

One of the next issues was finding an isolation room in the practice, which, like many local GPs' surgeries, was in an old house that had been adapted over the years. The only room that was suitable was the upstairs toilet. The bathroom was hastily decommissioned and reconfigured into an assessment unit for Covid. 'We were conscious, you didn't want to send every patient into hospital and burden the A&E departments. We did our best, and I wouldn't normally treat a patient in a toilet,' he says.

Ó Faoláin was soon inundated with calls – often as many as seventy or eighty every day. Patients grew frustrated at the lines jamming and, as many GPs will attest, the practice staff bore the brunt of panic and anger. 'They took all the abuse and kept showing up to work every day,' Ó Faoláin says. Due to the volume of calls, he set up an online call-back system. If a patient needed a Covid assessment, they could log their details and he would phone them back. His phone bill, usually around €200 per month, ballooned to €1,700.

'We were hit really bad in Ashbourne in March,' he says. 'We had about five or six deaths. A lot of men in their early fifties, previously healthy, ended up in ICU too.' Ó Faoláin thought this was the experience everywhere. He shared it on a GPs' WhatsApp group and people began to console him and urge him to take care of himself. 'I was thinking, "Is this not what everyone is experiencing?"'

In Dr Mary Favier's practice in Cork City, the ability of the GPs to serve as the 'canaries in the coalmine', rooting out what was really happening in the community, was becoming apparent. Dr Favier had seen a major upswing in Covid patients in late March and into early April. Presentations were not always the typical fever or shortness of breath medics had been told to be on the lookout for. 'What surprised us most was how variable the symptoms would be. There was a lot of time wasted in the beginning with the idea that it was just another version of the flu,' she says. 'The loss of taste and smell, which didn't become an official symptom until well into the summer, we were able to tell that was linked to Covid a long time back. It was something you got with Covid that you didn't get with anything else. It's what's called pathognomonic in medicine.'

Not all doctors saw an initial surge in calls. Some regions escaped the worst of the earliest days of the pandemic. Dr Amy Morgan, a GP in Drogheda, County Louth, says that things were eerily silent at first. This was initially a relief, but it became apparent that people were avoiding coming forward. She had to seek out patients, calling them to check in on them. 'Some people were actually sitting on quite worrying symptoms,' she says. 'They'd say, "Yeah, I've had a chest pain and I didn't want to be saying it to anybody."' Trying to gently nudge people in the direction of the hospital was a fearful prospect for so many of her patients. 'They were incredibly reluctant. People were just absolutely petrified.'

This experience was replicated at surgeries across the country, prompting many doctors to worry about what might go undiagnosed or unscreened, buried beneath the urgent need to address the rampage of the virus. As time wore on, the grim reality became unavoidable.

Morgan will always remember the first notification from hospital that one of her patients had died. She had looked after that patient and their family and knew them personally. The death was a difficult one to process. 'It seems obvious,' she says, 'you were turning on the news just like everybody else every day. You know people are dying of this. But in a way you nearly think your patients will be different. It was devastating. It was just so black and white.' A fax came through from the hospital about the cause of death. There were no comforting words or anything to hold on to. Just a sheet of paper. 'It just really crystallized it for me.'

There is no time to pause as a GP in this situation. Not in a pandemic. There is no time to contemplate or consider taking a morning off. 'You're having to tell your colleague about it and then the phones start hopping again because it's nine o'clock on a Tuesday morning.' It's an instant gear switch for family doctors. 'If someone is ringing about a mole that they're worried about, that's the most important thing to them. Even things that might seem trivial to other people, they're very real and they're important. All of a sudden it's, "okay, now we're talking about a rash."'

At times, Morgan would come home from the day worried about her patients and phone one or two of them to check in on them. It's hard to settle when things are so acute. When patients are frightened to go near a hospital or the GP practice itself. Often, she wouldn't talk about her day to her husband, trying to switch off by watching something on television. Other times, she'd click into webinars organized with GPs. Those provided a cathartic sense of unity. There were others who were going through the same situation. 'We rallied around each other,' she says; on WhatsApp group chats and weekly ICGP (Irish College of General Practitioners) webinars, 'We learned from each other. Everyone was really there for each other. I know it sounds corny but everyone was working together and trying to get through this.'

* * * *

The sense of 'we're all in this together' was also carefully crafted at a political level. Briefings with opposition leaders and health spokespeople were regular. Minister Simon Harris often fielded calls from Sinn Féin's Mary Lou McDonald, finding them helpful and supportive; political differences didn't enter the equation. It was stressed to politicians like the Social Democrats' Róisín Shortall and Labour's Alan Kelly at these briefings that they could be the Health Minister in a matter of weeks if a Government was formed. Micheál Martin deferred to his party's health spokesperson, Stephen Donnelly, who 'lectured us at great length', according to one health source. Róisín Shortall, herself a former Junior Health Minister who had worked on some level with Dr Tony Holohan, led a round of applause for the CMO at the first opposition briefing organized by the Department of Health.

The closest link struck up across party lines was between Harris and the Fianna Fáil leader, Micheál Martin. The pair built a close rapport. Harris had cleared the contacts with Leo Varadkar and ended up speaking to Martin almost every day, often more than that. Martin had a keen interest in public health and chimed in with his views on matters from face coverings to playgrounds to the St Patrick's Day parades. The political unity of purpose, and a post-election ceasefire, allowed the coalition to reframe itself.

Communications guru John Concannon, the creative force behind the Gathering initiative and the head of the scrapped and heavily criticized Special Communications Unit under Leo Varadkar's pre-election government, was brought back to the fold to mastermind the public awareness campaign. This was not an easy fit. The arrival of a spin doctor behind a €5m controversy, that Varadkar had been forced to concede was a 'distraction from the work of government' just two years earlier, was treated with suspicion by people within government.

Privately, the Departments of Health and the Taoiseach clashed over one of his proposals, which would have seen the CMO and NPHET press conferences moved from the Department of Health to the newly furnished press centre at Government Buildings. Senior officials in Health worried about the idea of having Tony Holohan's perceived independence stymied by getting him to present 'some sort of razzmatazz event every night with glitz and glamour and flashy videos'. Senior officials in Miesian Plaza were very concerned.

It was decided between Holohan and Simon Harris early on that there would be no political representation at the NPHET briefings. This would purely be public health advice offered by experts, unburdened by any political pressure. The idea was always that the NPHET press conference would be 'raw' and honest. 'There'll be shit news to deliver, there'll be good news on occasion. There will be times when they're a punching bag and a focal point for frustrations but they need to be independent,' says one former Health figure. 'I think the John Concannon thing was a disaster,' is the view of one minister who knew about the plan.

The view from the Government's civil service was that communications would be needed like never before. This would be 'Comms on Speed'. Pronouncements would be needed on public health messaging, explaining restrictions, schools, and more besides. Who else to turn to but this 'Wizard of Oz' who had successfully led marketing operations for the Gathering and the 1916 Centenary commemorations?

Liz Canavan from the Taoiseach's department appeared for near-daily press briefings at Government Buildings. Journalists at the briefings were not permitted to ask questions – bar an off-the-record briefing with officials after which could not be recorded – which two ministers have compared to 'North Korean newscasts': 'A government official reads out: 'Today is sunny and the Government is working hard on your behalf. Wash your hands. Government will mind you.'

* * * *

As the country found itself gripped by fear, it set about learning the new routines of working from home, social distancing

106

and organizing childcare for young students taken out of school. As Dr Catherine Motherway, intensive care consultant at University Hospital Limerick, drove home to the public on *Prime Time* – 'We need to treat each other like pariahs. Ideally, you don't need to get to see me. You need not to get this disease and you do that by keeping away from other people – two metres away, stay in your own home, wash your hands.'

The lockdown was hard for young families separated by continent, country, county or even a pane of glass. In a photograph that went viral around the world, Mícheál Ó Gallachóir showed off his new-born son Faolán to his dad Michael through the front window of his home in north Meath. To the world it was an emotional, heart-warming moment in our universal lockdown. To Mícheál and Emma Ó Gallachóir, it was a strange moment that typified a head-spinning few days. When Emma went into labour on Friday 13 March, the country was almost normal. The shops were open. People were out in cars on the roads. When she came out of hospital, Drogheda was a ghost town. The Ó Gallachóirs, in the space of three days, found themselves in an opened time capsule, as if a whole epoch had passed in the space of a mere three days. 'Faolán was born a week early. If he had been born on his due date, even a couple of days later, I would have been in there by myself,' says Emma.

When they came home, the traditional support bubble of grandparents and brothers and sisters who had kids of their own had evaporated. Nobody but Emma and Mícheál held Faolán for the first fifteen weeks of his life. All the advice, all the titbits of knowledge and support were delivered on the family WhatsApp or through the lens of FaceTime. 'Even to kind of say, "that's normal" or "yes, mine would've had that",' says Emma. There were none of the usual calls to the door by well-wishers and neighbours. The public health nurse arrived in the first week for the heel prick test; after that the driveway was empty for weeks.

The day Mícheál's parents came to the window was bitter-sweet. Their first grandchild, kept apart from them by this new pandemic where everyone wanted to do the right thing. The photo, shared across the world on Twitter and featured on US TV shows like *Good Morning America* and *Dr Phil*, became emblematic as a snapshot in time of three generations of the Ó Gallachóirs, but the reality that followed was a burden of huge stress for the new parents. 'It was very difficult. My mam and sisters would have expected to be here to help. They knew exactly the help you need the first time you bring a baby into the world and they felt for me that I didn't have that.' There were positives too; Mícheál was off work and the young family wouldn't have had that special time together without the three months of lockdown.

It was summer by the time Faolán's grandparents could finally meet him in person. Michael, his granddad, held him as if he were a newborn. 'He was mad to get in the door,' says Mícheál. 'He dotes over Faolán anyway. It's like, "Jesus, he wasn't like this with us … Who is this guy?"'

The return of a support network to the family was a godsend, but the following months brought with them the organizational challenges that would dog hundreds of house-holds in the early months of the pandemic, and the long ones to follow. Cancelled appointments; restrictions on baby swimming lessons – where Faolán could meet other babies for the first time – after three classes; restrictions on non-essential goods. All brought their own share of difficulty. Emma pushed for extended maternity leave as the time came to reschedule the appointments cancelled by hospital and GP restrictions. At times the couple felt that a lack of young voices or young families around the Cabinet table was detrimental to situa-tions like their own.

They feared baby Faolán would be uncomfortable around new people when the time eventually came. 'A nurse, when we did get into hospital, told us a lot of babies were making strange but we were lucky with Faolán, he's very outgoing,' says Mícheál with relief.

'I'd love to have met new mothers and been able to share the experience, but that just wasn't meant to be,' says Emma.

Chapter 8: Nursing Homes

Sheila Murphy wasn't from Clonakilty but she became a part of the town's fabric. A nurse for many years, she often stayed with people, caring for them as they died, making sure they had someone with them in their final days. People in the town still stop her daughters on the street to tell them how special she was, how amazing she was with older people. She nursed in Clonakilty Community Hospital, too, all the way through the 1980s. In April 2020, Sheila Murphy was one of ten people to die in a coronavirus outbreak at the hospital's care facility, where she had lived for the previous three years.

She was a city girl in her youth, a doctor's daughter who decided to pursue a vocation in nursing. The family still think Conor Murphy was strangely blessed when his car overturned after hitting a rock out at The Pike. He broke both legs and ended up in hospital, and Sheila Cronin was there to mind him. Conor was nearly thirty-three, Sheila was twenty-nine. They felt so lucky to have found each other and over the next six years they had six children. Sheila's daughters, Claire and Mary, sons Conor, Declan, Michael (Mary's twin) and John, and her beloved husband, Conor, doted on her.

As coronavirus appeared on the horizon in early 2020, however, the family feared the worst. There was a sense of helplessness as the far-off threat in January came first to Italy and then arrived on Ireland's shores at the end of February.

110

The first relief they felt since the turn of the year came with the Taoiseach's address in Washington: 'Finally, people will start to take this serious.'

The first warning came at the beginning of April. The Murphys were contacted by Clonakilty Community Hospital on 4 April; a staff member, on night duty on the first, had tested positive for Covid and a number of their colleagues had been forced out of work as close contacts. On the morning of 6 April, Claire and her father had a WhatsApp video call with a nurse in An Ghraig Ward who was able to connect Sheila and Conor by video. The nurse helped Sheila along as she sang to Conor, 'You are my sunshine, my only sunshine.' It was their last conversation, the last time they would see each other.

Days later another call from the hospital confirmed that there had been a positive test among the residents. Sheila's room, which she shared with three other people, was one of three multi-occupancy rooms in An Ghraig ward. Sheila had a high temperature, and was due to be tested the following day. Sheila's bed neighbour in An Ghraig was the first resident to test positive for the disease.

Claire Murphy called hour after hour trying to get through, looking for any kind of reassurance to offer her siblings, spread around the world, on the family WhatsApp. Mary, Claire's sister, was allowed in to visit and could see that things were challenging. 'I was allowed to go in one day and it was like going into a war zone. It was scary in there. In the room where my mom was dying there were two televisions and the telephone and there was loads of noise. Mom got her test and she tested positive. I think we kind of knew it was coming and my question was: What do we do now?' She asked what arrangements were in place. Would Sheila be transferred to ICU if she became very sick? Were there ventilators in place? Was there morphine?

Claire had struck up a strong relationship with the staff nurse on call. She knew the best time to call and, using the knowledge passed down over the years by Sheila, the right questions to ask. Claire would call at 7 a.m. to catch the switchover of night and day shifts, at 7 p.m. to catch the next changeover, and at 11 p.m. just so she could give her dad an update on how his wife was doing before he went to sleep. It was a routine that continued for days. Conor anxious to hear about Sheila, the Murphy siblings in Cork and around the world desperate too for information, looking at their screens at all hours of the day waiting to hear any news that things might be changing for the better.

They agonized for a time as to whether or not they should have brought Sheila home, just as so many other families did. It was impossible. 'We knew we couldn't bring her home,' says Claire. 'Even though we wished we could, it just wasn't going to be an option.' When Sheila tested positive for Covid, Claire filled the house with photos of her, giving herself and her dad the chance to reminisce and talk about sweet memories of their lives together.

The calls continued, becoming harder to hear as nurses' voices became muffled through masks. The calls with Sheila's nurse almost reminded them of Sheila in a way; the Murphys would remember her coming home from night duty after sitting with people as they died.

On Saturday the nineteenth, Claire rang for her dad's 11 p.m. update. 'Now, your report for your dad is that your mum is very comfortable and she's resting and she'll have a good night's sleep,' the nurse said. 'And now for you,' she said to Claire. 'Make sure you have your phone with you when you go to bed and that your dad won't hear it because I will phone you before the morning because your mum won't see the morning.'

It is not a phone call any daughter or son wants to hear about their parent. In the first wave, more than a thousand lives were lost to the virus in nursing homes and long-term care facilities. These calls are forever seared into the memory of countless families across the country. No one who received one will ever forget where they were or what time of the day it was when they were called.

Claire's phone rang again at 4.30 a.m. Sheila didn't have much longer. The final call came at 5.07 a.m. Sheila had died at 5.05. The nurses had stayed with her. They said the Rosary with her. They talked about her darling Conor, and their six wonderful children and eight beloved grandchildren. Sheila always said that if someone was struggling to die, it was important to let them know that the people they loved would be okay and it was safe for them to go. The nurses told them they had done this by Sheila's bedside in her final moments.

Claire hung up the phone, sitting on the bed in a daze. It was too early to tell her dad. She called the hospital back. 'What do I do now?' she asked. She was told that it was her role to ring the undertaker, who would work with the hospital. Sheila Murphy was buried within twelve and a half hours of her death.

The Murphys discussed whether or not to do something in the church, just across the street from them on Western Road in Clonakilty town. There were storage issues at the undertakers and at the hospital. At noon, the panicked undertaker called to say that the Monsignor could organize a mass between then and the evening.

'The best thing, Dad felt, and we all felt anyway, she didn't need any more masses,' says Mary. 'I think as well, Dad didn't want to be in the church with a coffin he hadn't closed. He didn't want to be sitting there with the coffin with Sheila's remains in it if he hadn't seen her. It would have been too hard.' The coming hours were traumatic. At midday, the undertaker rang Claire to say that 'the hospital didn't have anywhere for Sheila so I had to remove her'.

'I just remember when Charles, the undertaker, said "I have your mother and I have her somewhere safe." I said, "You mean she's in the back of the hearse in your yard?" and he didn't say no but just said again "I have her somewhere safe."' Claire says, 'Charles was crying that day. I guess undertakers don't cry very easily. He was certainly crying that day.'

Declan Murphy in Brunei had contacted a family friend, musician Ger Wolfe, to record a song for Sheila, and Cork soprano Fiona O'Reilly recorded one of her favourite pieces, 'Que Sera'. Everyone who knew she was going to the grave was out on the street that morning to see her off. The Murphys met Sheila's remains at the churchyard and drove as far as their house. 'We just walked up with the coffin,' Mary says. The undertaker worried that a crowd would form as others saw the family make their way. They stayed where they were, standing respectfully to mourn someone who had made such a difference to the town.

There have been many notes to Conor and the family since Sheila's passing thanking him for bringing this force of nature to Clonakilty. Everyone who came across her loved her and was inspired by her sense of justice. 'She was a fair bit of a socialist,' Mary laughed, 'and well able to argue with anyone about politics.'

Sheila had been raised in an egalitarian household, her dad a GP, 'a scholarship boy'. All six of her sisters sat the Leaving Cert in the 1940s and 50s. When Conor's family met her they said, 'He's marrying a doctor's daughter', but as Sheila used to tell her own children, 'They didn't understand what kind of a doctor's daughter I was.' She fought many a battle and raised her children to be empathetic. Coming home off night duty, to discover the house was like a bomb site, she'd stand in the kitchen singing Bob Marley's 'Get up, stand up, stand up for your rights' to Mary and her twin brother when they were teenagers, making sure they understood that they'd need to pull their weight and couldn't expect her to come home to a tip after a long night of work.

Sheila had found an image of the scales of justice on the internet, printing it out and attaching it to postcards she made to send to members of the Government calling for action on various issues. Ringing politicians to register her upset. Enda Kenny's WhatsApp is still on Claire's phone from one of Sheila's many campaigns to try to convince people to do the right thing. Over the years, one of her most successful drives was writing to make sure widows denied their pensions were properly reimbursed. One wonders what she would have made of the pandemic and its impact on the most vulnerable.

Mary and Claire have looked after their dad Conor, going on walks or for drives with him. Months later, pulling in after a spin through the estuary and past the picturesque piers of Ring, Conor cried, tears pouring down his face. 'I just miss her so much but I'm so glad I met her.'

The Murphys addressed a number of queries to Clonakilty Community Hospital about Sheila's care in April 2020. The hospital responded that they 'would be willing to sit down when the time is right'. The family replied, 'We appreciate the fact that we will be able to sit down with you in the future to get answers to these questions. We're not letting you off the hook.'

One thing the Murphys have said is that individual staff members on the frontline at the Community Hospital were stellar, going above and beyond for Sheila and to do what was right by her. One quick-thinking staff member, when Sheila died, went up to her room. She grabbed a photo of Sheila and Conor, a knitted bunny comforter the family had made for her and a crucifix. She put them with Sheila before she was removed. The staff member had turned up to the grave-yard multiple times and waited, to try to catch the family, not knowing where they lived. They wanted Conor to know. 'I was doing it, because it needed to be done,' they said.

The Murphys are glad that Sheila is at peace now. But it pains them to think of the time that was taken from them.

Sheila was tactile. Touch was so close to the essence of who she was as a mother and a person. 'If anyone was upset, she'd rub your head, she'd rub your face, she'd hold your hand. To not be able to touch her is heart-breaking,' says Mary. 'Loads of people I would have considered friends made such flippant remarks about, "Oh sure, it's only people in their eighties." Yeah, these are all people who hadn't a long time left but they would have died in a way that didn't leave this gaping hole in families. Sometimes I'd feel like screaming out: "You don't know what it's like to lose your mom to this. It's different."'

Some people around town whispered: 'Well, at least the virus isn't here.' Mary says in response to them: 'There are several people dying in the hospital. The market is full of people every week who've moved here because Clon is cool. But Clon is cool because of the octogenarians who stayed and who made it. There were ten or eleven people who died in a ten-day period who were from in and around Clonakilty. That's a horrendous loss of people from a small town.'

Claire and Mary's interview was done over Zoom. It's a painful experience to join two siblings, both suffering the pain of loss in a pandemic, separated across two different households. 'We can't even hug each other, you know?' says Claire. 'Like that's my only sister, my baby sister, and all I want to do all year is to hold her and hug her and we can't. We're afraid to do that even, you know. It's important to remember everyone who died this year was a human being. I do think Sheila was a very exceptional human being but they were all people. It's important to remember that.'

* * * *

A Health Information and Quality Authority (HIQA) report into Clonakilty Community Hospital found that the facility hadn't adhered to Covid guidelines during the outbreak there in April and May. Its inspection report from June told how residents who had been in close contact, or who were suspected of being infected, or who were known to be infected, were not moved to isolation or quarantine.

Multi-occupancy bedrooms, the watchdog said, had a 'significant impact' on how the outbreak was managed, and concerns about rooms had been raised years in advance of the outbreak, in five earlier inspection reports going back to March 2017, and in three meetings with HSE management.

The HSE responded to the report saying that residents who tested positive remained in shared bedrooms with others who may have previously tested negative or were not showing symptoms and that this was due to the limitations of the physical premises.

* * * *

Many nursing homes suffered unthinkable loss of life from Covid-19 in the spring of 2020. Forty people died at Ryevale Nursing Home in Leixlip, County Kildare. Twenty-nine died in Marymount Care Centre in Lucan, County Dublin. Twenty-three people died at Dealgan House in Dundalk, County Louth, where the private nursing home was temporarily taken over by the Royal College of Surgeons in Ireland hospital group to manage the outbreak.

Many families of those who died have come together to call for a public inquiry into what happened in these, and other, nursing homes during Covid-19. They feel that preparations were not made early enough. That the PPE was not adequately available. That infection control in some facilities was not rigid enough. That the transfer of patients, assessed but untested, from acute hospitals to nursing homes in the spring of 2020 was a risk that may have introduced infection to homes.

The authorities and the Government, in defending the

response to nursing homes, say that all the early focus at the time was on avoiding a Bergamo situation; the threat of overloaded ICUs and broken hospitals was too much to bear at the time. A laser-like focus on the frontline of healthcare was the overriding characteristic of the early State response. While the Taoiseach had mentioned the need for older people to cocoon in their homes in his St Patrick's Day speech, there was no mention at that point of nursing homes.

Tadhg Daly is the CEO of Nursing Homes Ireland (NHI), the representative group for the owners of private nursing homes. In the early days of the pandemic, he had no sense that the situation in care facilities would become so ferocious. There was engagement with the Department of Health on PPE stocks, Daly anxiously noting how the HSE had made clear in the media there would be 'adequate stock', with the majority to be focused on primary care and GP surgeries. However, 'This is not the case for our member nursing homes,' Daly said in an email to the Department. 'The level of indifference towards the sector was striking,' he says.

Much of the focus on nursing homes comes from the early guidance on visitor restrictions. On 6 March, NHI issued a directive. 'No non-essential visiting, children or groups will be allowed' according to the notice; 'visitors should only seek to attend in urgent circumstances and the management reserve the right to impose full restrictions where necessary.' Daly was on his way to Dublin and speaking to government officials on the phone, who were asking him to hold off on issuing the directive. He felt it was the right decision to make.

That evening, at NPHET's press briefing, Tony Holohan pushed back: 'We ask that no organization, school or health service provider acts unilaterally. We need to respond to the threat of Covid-19 in unison, following the advice of Public Health.' The CMO's view was upheld at NPHET's meeting on 10 March, the minutes of which show: 'It was agreed that the current practice of restricting visitors to nursing homes was not required and this would be kept under review.'

Within two days, it would be reviewed, when Ireland entered its first social restrictions on 12 March. Holohan, NPHET and the HSE say that the picture had changed rapidly. The number of new infections was rising fast. Embers of community spread of the virus were sparking and would soon turn into an inferno.

Nursing homes were already feeling the pressure. Staff at one facility in the east of the country raised their concerns in direct messages with me on Twitter about families coming in to visit relatives after stopping off in the shops, taking their bags with them. One nurse said she was 'shaking' after seeing people walk in and out with no apparent regard for social distancing or the infection control measures visitors were informed about on arrival.

Paul Reid of the HSE says an early row with NPHET and Dr Tony Holohan came over this delay on visitor restrictions. 'That was the first kind of mode of conflict between the Public Health guys and our guys because I defended the nursing homes taking decisions to stop the visitors. I defended the nursing homes curtailing or restricting visitors, whereas Tony had said they shouldn't have done that, you know. And they should, you know?'

Holohan's defence of his nursing home intervention points to the fact that the vast majority of new infections and clusters in nursing homes came more than two weeks after the re-imposition of visitor restrictions on 13 March.

In any case, what did follow in the nursing homes was the most devastating impact of the uncontrolled spread of the virus in confined settings, preying on vulnerable people, and a staff who, in many cases, simply did not have the means to cope with it. By 29 March, there were twenty-four clusters of infection in Ireland's nursing homes. A month later, there were 219. The situation was out of control.

The State's capacity to test crumpled under the weight of demand. A HSE memo on 21 March from David Walsh, the National Director of Community Operations, to the HSE's Community Healthcare Organisations read: 'Following confirmation of a Covid positive diagnosis within the unit/centre then it is assumed that all residents presenting with symptoms are Covid positive. Multiple re-referrals to NAS for potential Covid cases should be avoided.'

It was not until 17 April that mass testing could be carried out for all residents and staff of long-term residential care facilities.

The glow of a St Patrick's Day well done had worn off Richard Quinlan of the National Ambulance Service. The nursing home crisis was now the top priority for his crews. 'There's something not right here,' Richard thought in late March as he listened to the radio news en route between jobs and as the situation in care homes became clear. 'This isn't going well.' In early April, the NAS was instructed that mass swabbing at nursing homes would be its prime focus.

The NAS couldn't swab everyone on its own. The closure of elective and ancillary services across Irish healthcare saw staff from all backgrounds redirected to what was becoming a national effort of heightening urgency. Specialists from orthopaedics, ophthalmology, dentistry and facial reconstruction were among the teams put together, which included Defence Forces medics and Community First Responders.

Every morning, Quinlan stood in the yard at Cherry Orchard ambulance station to address the motley crew of specialists and volunteers. The teams stood looking back at him, some carrying phone chargers and plastic bags of extra food they'd need for the day. Everyone knew what was being asked of them and how desperate the situation had become. Nobody was under any illusion as to what they would face over the course of the coming hours. The briefings would all begin the same way – with a readout of the swabs completed over the previous day's work and the latest positivity percentage to be fed back from the labs and regional public health teams.

Once the teams had been given coffee and pastries, they set off together in convoys. Fourteen-seat minibuses were hired, with six people sitting in each, socially distanced. Two or three buses plus ambulances would arrive at a nursing home, assess the site and get down to work. Anywhere between 5,000 and 7,000 swabs would be collected across twelve-hour days in Dublin and north Leinster. That effort was replicated by the crews across the country.

For the intensity of mass-swabbing to work, it had to be blanket. 'Everyone from the gate in gets swabbed,' was the rule. Richard Quinlan got a call from one team swabbing at a nursing home in Leinster, 'There are two undertakers here to remove bodies.' 'Swab them,' was his instant response. It was a horrifying scene for the team on the ground. As they were arriving to help resolve the situation, two undertakers retrieving two bodies were trying to leave. This was the bare face of Covid in nursing homes. Cruel. Relentless. Punishing.

People were dying. The gravity of the situation was clear to everyone involved and was a difficult burden to carry. Many facilities were on their knees, long past the point of rescue. At one stage, an exhausted Quinlan got a late-night call. He was back in the Green Isle Hotel after a long day of swabbing, his mind thinking back to the distress of the homes they'd recently worked in. A geriatrician in one of the HSE task forces called him in a panic – staff had gone down in one facility. They were all positive and there was no one to man the place. 'Can you help?'

The images from nursing homes in Spain where soldiers sent to assist disinfection found whole corridors of older people dead, abandoned by staff, were vivid in Quinlan and his crews' minds. 'This is really, really bad,' says Richard, haunted by the

121

experience. 'You're having these conversations and you think "I can see the next step here if we're not careful."'

Two ambulances went out to take control of the home. Retired staff volunteered to cover the shift. The worried, whispered phone calls continued through the night. The hours seemed unending. Walking the corridors, the NAS crews were shattered, looking around at the Covid posters and listening to the shifting and groans overnight. Quinlan and local public health teams were petrified by the situation. 'I don't want this to be in the news tomorrow,' he thought. Nothing in basic training covered this. At daybreak, relief staff arrived. This was just another aspect of many in the nursing homes context where a desperate situation teetered on the brink of another scale of catastrophe entirely.

The PPE crisis pushed many homes to take desperate measures. One facility, responding to an NHI study, resorted to using 'painters' overalls, painters' goggles, surgical masks that cost €1.50 each'. Another was donated goggles from a local school, gowns from a local vet and masks made by a local dressmaker. There were facilities across the country where staff who had seen colleagues and residents become infected were forced to reuse aprons, goggles and masks far beyond their single-use intention. The anxiety was crippling.

One memo from the HSE in the Midlands in mid-April said PPE 'should only be used for confirmed/suspect client cases and not for normal use within the services'. This, to Tadhg Daly's mind, was 'inappropriate' and amounted to a rationing of PPE in the most desperate of circumstances.

The wait for testing became so long that it was almost redundant in some homes. Nursing home staff who have spoken to me detailed experiences of waiting three weeks for swabs, with results often coming in after residents had died. One nursing home director, speaking about how in mid-April several residents had died in their facility, recalled ringing Tadhg Daly late at night to vent about the situation. 'It was horrific. I couldn't comprehend what was happening. I was really, really upset by it. I couldn't comprehend what was happening inside. People were dying, staff were out sick. It was traumatizing. I have no other word for it.'

In early April, HIQA's Chief Inspector of Social Services Mary Dunnion told the Department of Health that sixty-seven per cent of nursing homes were not compliant with care and welfare regulations, and that 124 public and private nursing homes, a quarter of the total in Ireland, were at risk and needed additional HSE support. HIQA maintains that it has never been given enough power to move quickly when it detects instances of non-compliance, an issue it raised with both Minister Simon Harris and his successor. HIQA inspectors found the impact on staff in nursing homes one of the most upsetting elements of their work. Some staff left because of illness; some never came back. A HIQA report detailing the experience of nursing homes in the first wave found that, in many situations, 'routine infection prevention and control measures were not being followed'. One nursing home 'left bedroom doors open for residents that had tested positive'; in another 'staff were observed caring for residents in close proximity without using surgical masks'; in some cases 'temperature checks on staff were not being documented'.

At Dealgan House in County Louth, where twenty-three people died with Covid-19, Dolores Conroy, the home's assistant director of nursing, told *The Pat Kenny Show* on Newstalk how the virus and a lack of external support had left staff struggling with post-traumatic stress disorder. In April, she said, 'Everybody knew we were in crisis. HIQA was asked for help. I begged them for help on April the sixth. I was not only managing the nursing home, I was also a nurse with no management in the building.'

Conroy's experience was chillingly familiar at homes across the country. Staff were forced to fight on through fourteen-hour days or longer, seeing their colleagues fall sick to disease and residents they'd known for years die.

'The staff were hysterical here during the deaths because some days we had two deaths. Some people had no symptoms and just went to sleep and never woke up.

'Staff are still struggling with the after-effects, with panic attacks, with post-traumatic stress, and some of our staff still have post-viral symptoms even now after having the Covid.'

Nursing home owners are, to this day, angered by what they deem the 'poaching' of senior nursing staff from their positions by the HSE in the early days of the pandemic. It's a practice of 'robbing Peter to pay Paul', in the view of NHI's Tadhg Daly. The sense of crisis in some nursing homes was worsened by the absence of key management staff who had left to take up roles in the acute sector. Nursing home providers remain dissatisfied with the transfer of patients to nursing homes in the spring of 2020. Many still believe they were a key source of infection introduced into the homes. However, as previously mentioned, NPHET says the timing of the surge in nursing homes came many weeks after the imposition of restrictions in nursing homes. Tony Holohan remains adamant transfers were not the cause of the devastation.

'The easiest thing for me to say would be that it's terrible, the HSE should have moved quicker on mass testing,' says one senior official, 'but they were really trying. It was frustrating how long it was taking to get things done but the real issue is the model of care. The actual thing we could have done better is cared for older people properly before the pandemic arrived. Why, when I reach seventy, do I have to pack my bags and move out of my community and into some kind of large house and live with a load of other people?'

Staff involved in the State's response bear the emotional scars of the nursing home crisis. 'I find it hard to talk about,' says one, 'it's emotional now. Once it got into the nursing homes there was genuinely no way of stopping it. And that was the hardest part because, you know, almost all of the time it came in through the staff, most of whom were foreign nationals who were living in congregated settings themselves.'

Holohan says the world didn't have the same sense about the 'particular risk' this virus posed for older people, especially in congregated sectors and in nursing homes. 'From previous pandemics, the focus might not have been so much on that particular sector. From our point of view, the whole thing was about getting community transmission down. We knew that widespread community transmission was a threat to everybody and to everything. We had no chance of protecting anywhere if the disease is ripping through the population at large. All the way through March, the measures were interventions aimed at minimizing that and that's what you have to do to protect workplaces or schools or nursing homes.'

Simon Harris, all but living in the Department of Health at the time, his wife working as a nurse in a children's hospital, was FaceTiming residents of nursing homes, hearing first hand about the fear they had. Some people used to cry on the calls, becoming overwhelmed about not being able to see their family members except through a window.

The criticism of the State's response is unlikely to lift until there has been a full inquiry. Leo Varadkar admits that the focus on the hospitals was the number one priority for the Government in the early days of the pandemic. He doesn't regret it. 'It was the right decision,' he says, based on what was happening in Italy and Spain. Even if the Government had known the nursing homes would become ground zero for the crisis, he says, there would be little opportunity to fortify them. 'We wouldn't have been able to invent up staff that didn't exist or PPE that we didn't have or get testing in there quicker. I don't honestly think we could have resolved those issues.'

The matter was brought home to each member of the

Government in different ways. On Easter weekend, Justice Minister Charlie Flanagan looked out of his window in Portlaoise and witnessed hearse after hearse rumbling up the grit road, leaving a local care facility. Eight people died over the long weekend in a nursing unit 250 yards from his home. 'It was scary. The horror of what happened. I saw the hearses actually pass up the road, individual hearses with nobody around and that was chilling. That to me was the darkest hour.'

Not everyone at Cabinet believes the government response was good enough. One Fine Gael minister, heavily involved in the early response to the pandemic, says of the nursing homes: 'They were in total disarray and screaming for help. I have to think that we were ignoring them. I don't know this for sure, but it just looked like we weren't stepping up to the plate, probably because we were in our own disarray, but it did take too long.' The facility in the minister's hometown was flattened by the virus. 'Their staff just fell away, because they were either sick, or just weren't coming to work out of fear. We should have went there first. It was the older, vulnerable people with underlying conditions who were the most at risk.

'They're Irish citizens and we had a responsibility to them and I don't think we were fast enough.' The minister says it wasn't any one Department's fault or any one minister's fault, but it is 'wrong' that the nursing homes weren't an immediate priority. 'Looking at the pleas and cries from all of the individual nursing homes, it didn't look like they were being heeded for probably too long.'

The minister points to St Mary's in the Phoenix Park and the devastating outbreak there. 'They were screaming [for help], and that was a HSE-run nursing home. So, if we weren't looking after the nursing homes that were being run and managed by the health service, I think that tells you that we didn't get to the private nursing homes until it was too late for some of the people who passed away.'

Chapter 9: Stolen Goodbyes

'Are you okay?'

The garda leaned forward to look in the window. Catherine Lawlor was not okay. She was wrecked, exhausted beyond her limits. She had been stopped at a Covid checkpoint on the N7, perhaps her third of the journey since leaving the Phoenix Park. She just wanted to go home. Tears were streaming down her face. She wasn't able to talk. Her mind was racing all that way home: 'I'm afraid. Have I got *it*?' She'd changed her clothes, she'd showered, but she just didn't know for certain.

She flashed her healthcare worker badge in the direction of the garda without saying a word. He was immediately apologetic: 'Oh my God, are you okay?'

Catherine had had enough. Saying nothing, she continued her journey. The Clinical Nursing Manager at St Mary's had been through another day of fear and grief at work. This was not normal.

St Mary's Hospital in the Phoenix Park, run by the HSE, is one of the country's largest nursing homes, home to around one hundred and fifty residents. It's a home that, in normal times, is a happy place, with organized outings, music, bingo and art classes. The communal rooms are often characterized by great laughter and chats, with staff all too happy to spend hours encouraging residents to reminisce and bring out their memories with old photos of Dublin 'in the rare auld times'.

As the month of March 2020 rolled on, the music fell silent. The St Patrick's Day concert, a highlight of the year, was cancelled and residents grew concerned about news of the virus. The staff did too. St Mary's soon found itself at the centre of one of the worst losses of life in the first wave of the Covid-19 pandemic.

The first case was confirmed on 28 March, with the outbreak at its worst across the long month of April. The fear had long set in by then, the laughter of old giving way to quiet terror among residents. 'Some residents asked staff "Will I get it?"' says Catherine Lawlor. 'You'd walk into a room and people were terrified.' The best thing to do in those situations is to relate. Catherine and her colleagues did their best to reassure people, explaining that they too were terrified. 'It was awful. I'll never forget the fear.'

Rosie Hegarty knew nursing homes would be in trouble. The eighty-four-year-old from Finglas was well abreast of the Covid-19 news, reading stories about care homes in Seattle and Spain, and the devastation being wrought on vulnerable communities as staff, in some instances, walked off the job. Her niece, Jane Carrigan, remembers Rosie watching Taoiseach Leo Varadkar's speech from Washington, DC on 12 March, in which he announced the first restrictions. Such was Rosie's appetite for news, she would get frustrated when Jane and her sister Cathy called without any news to tell her. This meant the two sisters would have to tic-tac their calls so they always alternated.

Rosie had already taken her own precautions against Covid. Even in early February, when she had to attend an outpatient appointment at Beaumont Hospital, she went through weeks of debate with her family about whether or not it was safe for her to go in. In the end she went, accompanied by a tall member of St Mary's staff. Rosie got a kick out of being one of the few people in the hospital that day – 'little old me in the wheelchair and my six-foot chaperone!'

Back at St Mary's, she insisted on staying in her room. This was no major issue for her. She had a love of nature, and her ground floor window looked across the garden. Often the small herd of deer that stick to this sheltered corner of the Phoenix Park passed by her window, chewing the green grass outside. From early March, she skipped communal meals. Her food was brought to her room, which was at the end of a corridor. She felt safer there.

She loved life in St Mary's before the pandemic arrived. The organized activities both inside and outside the hospital were a huge hit with Rosie. She enjoyed taking part in the gardening club and going out to lunch with staff and her friends on occasion. At Christmas 2019, staff members took her to a shopping centre to buy Christmas presents. 'It was a new lease of life,' remembers Jane, who says Rosie had been withdrawing more and more from life in the ten years before she decided that St Mary's would be the home for her.

She was, in many ways, a larger-than-life character – a 'live wire'. One of her nieces' fondest memories of Rosie is during the 1990 World Cup. She adored football, and was as wrapped up in the national frenzy around Jack's Army as anyone in the country. Rosie was the sort of football fan who feared the worst. She feared the team would be destroyed over in Italy, but once they got to the second round, she promised she'd dye her hair green if they beat Romania. She was out in the driveway, pacing, unable to watch any of the match, but was as good as her word when David O'Leary's penalty sent the nation into raptures. It is this sense of fun, Jane says, that will always stay with them.

Rosie had a strong sense of social justice. Her appetite for news and politics was endless. In 2019, she was determined to get out of St Mary's in her wheelchair to protest Donald Trump's visit. Jane encouraged these plans but at the same time had a real fear that the two of them would get arrested, Rosie shouting all manner of things and Jane effectively the fall guy beside her. 'She had a huge interest in the life outside of her world, which now was getting smaller.'

With precautions in place from March, staff were preparing themselves for what was to come. They diligently watched the webinars on donning and doffing protective equipment, but by early April, there were concerns both about how much PPE was available and also when it should be used. In emails between staff and management, first published in the *Irish Times*, a member of staff at St Mary's said they were 'gravely concerned' about access to masks, gowns and other materials and when they should be used: 'If someone has one symptom, and we are not using PPE, there is an obvious risk that if the person does actually have Covid-19 we as front-line workers will get it and will be carriers, transmitting it to other residents.'

Families of some residents say they heard concerns expressed by staff about the provision of PPE gear in March and April. This would later become a real worry for many of them. As PPE supplies landed to fanfare in Dublin Airport, some staff privately wished they'd drive straight down the M50 and out to the Phoenix Park to St Mary's.

One healthcare assistant, Ruth, remembers the horror of being sent a photo by one of her colleagues, who was trying to protect herself with a paper towel over her mouth and nose because residents were 'coughing in her face'. Ruth, who later worked three shifts back to back over the course of seventy-two hours, left the building and sobbed heavy, breathless tears. 'It was sheer terror,' she says. 'I felt unprotected and unsafe, as did everybody to be honest with you. I didn't feel terrified of getting sick myself or even my family. My biggest fear was being a carrier and being the cause of someone else getting sick or causing a fatality or even multiple fatalities. That was my biggest fear.'

It is clear that the nature of the infections caught the hospital by surprise. All the early messaging to them had been focused on high fever, a temperature and respiratory symptoms such as a cough. For many older people in nursing homes like St Mary's and across the country, this was not how the virus presented itself.

Dr Chei Wei 'Mimi' Fan is a consultant geriatrician at the Mater Hospital and at St Mary's. She says that recognizing the virus was the problem. Staff would wear full PPE suits when there was a positive diagnosis of Covid, she says. But the problem was trying to get that diagnosis. 'I'd say most people caught it because the infection wasn't that well defined in the beginning,' she says. 'Now we are extra careful. I think if they were Covid positive, you would definitely have [full PPE]. It's just recognizing the disease to put on the stuff. The whole drive was to get the people protected and to protect the residents, to protect ourselves so that we can work.'

She remembers the first patient who was sent to hospital and later swabbed positive for Covid. He was 'strikingly drowsy', sleepy all the time. Mimi was looking after this man and had a hunch. She put on the full kit, just in case, and he was admitted to hospital for further assessment and treatment. His positive result was, for Mimi, the moment staff started to realize that perhaps this virus was presenting slightly differently in older people.

'They had the Covid but we didn't know, we were looking for temperatures,' says Catherine Lawlor. Residents who became sick were drowsy, or went off their food, 'everything tasted like cardboard' – perhaps it was their sense of taste and smell that had left them; others had pains or diarrhoea. The staff at St Mary's had followed the guidelines but were caught out by how the disease presented. If the different symptoms had been known sooner, many staff believe what was to follow could have been avoided.

The first case was confirmed on 28 March.

131

Getting positive results itself was a battle. Aisling Coffey is Principal Social Worker at St Mary's. A vibrant and cheerful person, she wears her heart on her sleeve, and her love for the facility, the staff and, most of all, the residents is clear. 'There were challenges throughout the system with getting prompt testing of older people and staff and getting prompt results back,' she says. She was one of many staff who were shocked to see the first confirmed case in the nursing home on site, rather than in the short-stay hospital which took admissions from the Mater.

Swabbing was not an easy task. Dr Fan says that people with dementia were distressed. Some didn't want to or couldn't open their mouths, with staff having to carefully hold their heads while swabs were taken from the nostril. It added to the challenge.

Jane Carrigan's sister Cathy was told on 29 March that there was a case in St Mary's. It was the family's worst fear, and they debated whether or not to tell Rosie. She had been taking extra care, making sure her room was well-ventilated and that sanitizer was always close at hand. But Rosie 'knew the beat of the nursing home', says Jane. Her nieces didn't have to tell her there was something going on. She'd seen extra activity, watching faces of new staff members move by her door, murmurs and noises and panicked expressions. She asked staff members what was happening and learned about the case. She phoned her nieces on the thirtieth, confirming what they'd already been told. The fact that the confirmed case was in another ward was a strange relief to them. 'You're thinking "Okay, this is awful and a tragedy but it's the far side of a really big building. Everything's still OK." We were just trying to plough away as normal but, really, we were on a countdown at that stage.'

They spoke to Rosie every single day. Hoping against hope that the virus wasn't closing in. Mental milestones were created – 'We'll just get through a week. Another week. We'll be in the clear.' But 'it didn't work out like that,' Jane says. 'The infection seemed to really go quite quickly through St Mary's.'

Healthcare assistant Ruth continued to work through her concerns about PPE, which she says was now being strictly rationed. On arrival into Oisin ward in early April, she says, masks were left out of boxes on tables and staff were given three masks each for the duration of the entire day. Coming in with one mask of her own, Ruth was only given two.

A whistleblower at the hospital, who later filed a protected disclosure, emailed management on 4 April outlining serious concerns about the movement of symptomatic patients between wards, the provision of PPE and whether or not residents with a single symptom were being treated as suspected cases.

She told them she was 'terrified' about possibly transmitting the disease unknowingly without proper PPE. She claimed that staff were not permitted to wear masks when around residents who had a cough but no fever, and that she was told to 'take a step back' if a patient coughed. The whistleblower told management a resident did accidentally cough directly into her face on the day she sent the email.

The concerns were not limited to the whistleblower; by now families were contacting journalists in panic, unable to get through to staff for updates on their family members. Other staff say there was one evening when masks weren't ready and healthcare assistants were told to hand out suppers into residents' rooms without proper protective equipment. 'We were told not to wear masks; I always refused not to. I was told to go in and hold a mobile phone to somebody's ear. I never did any of those things.'

By 17 April, eleven deaths had been confirmed in St Mary's. In a statement, the HSE expressed its sympathies to the friends and families of those who had died: 'our thoughts are with them at this difficult time. We remain in contact with relatives and next-of-kin of all residents within St Mary's Hospital in relation to any suspect or confirmed cases of Covid-19.'

An internal memo from the time showed evidence of 'more than 20 per cent' confirmed or suspected infection in St Mary's. 'It is reasonable to assume that transmission is generalized,' the memo said. 'The entire clinical area of the unit is designated a contaminated zone.' The memo, drafted following a visit by the HSE's Infection Prevention Control lead, Professor Martin Cormican, directed staff to set up 'clean' and 'dirty' areas, referring to residents with no symptoms as the 'cleanest', those with suspected cases as 'dirty' and those with confirmed Covid as 'dirtiest patients'.

This provoked fury from residents' families. 'To say that I am offended by this is an understatement,' said Dr Gerri O'Neill on Twitter. 'My relative is not "dirty".' The HSE was forced to express regret over the memo, which they said was issued in error without formal approval. Dr Colm Henry, Chief Clinical Officer, said that the language had 'no place' anywhere in medicine. Professor Cormican, cited in the memo, was furious about it. 'Someone wrote a memo and put my name on it,' he says. 'What people went through, both the residents and the staff, was extraordinarily difficult. They were shattered,' he says of the staff, 'and fragile. They needed support. I hope and certainly tried to frame anything I had to say as "here's how I think you could be doing better", rather than "here's what you're doing wrong".'

Professor Dermot Power, a consultant geriatrician at the Mater Hospital, was one of those brought in to help tackle the cluster. He told the *Irish Times* that the slow pace of test results made everything worse, leading to staff with colds being out unnecessarily, waiting for their Covid results – others, without symptoms but who had Covid, may have continued to work. It was the 'perfect storm', he said.

Heat made the staff's challenges all the more difficult.

While the photos used by most news organizations during the outbreak were of the gates or the old hospital building, the nursing home was based in two new units with large glass windows. The Phoenix Park's weather station recorded just 5.8 mm of rain between 18 March and 28 April. Nursing homes, by their nature, are warm. The sunshine, glaring through the windows, added to it. Nurses and HCAs in full PPE, effectively 'boiler suits' as one nurse put it, were faced with unbearable heat in some rooms and corridors that felt like glasshouses. 'The rooms get really hot,' says HCA Alison Fitzgerald. The hospital's facilities manager sent relays to fetch drinks and ice creams for staff, often working twelve-hour shifts in PPE. 'By the time you got to go for your lunch, you were exhausted. By the end of the day, you were exhausted.'

Measures were put in place to make sure that infection was minimized. Covid patients were assigned to one team of staff, non-Covid residents to another team. There was no switching of responsibilities or crossing over between wards.

The early lockdown weather brought families out to the park for picnics, bike rides and kickabouts, many of them on the vast lawn sloping down to the Chapelizod Road gate which is overlooked by the old St Mary's building. The serenity, even the novelty, of the early days of lockdown for some was worlds away from the grief and suffering in the building close by. Some staff often wondered if the people they'd pass arriving into work even knew they were there.

St Mary's is right beside the NAS base, so close in fact that you 'could hit it with a rock' in the words of Richard Quinlan, chief ambulance officer operating out of the base. What happened across the field from them over the coming weeks was a surreal and terrifying reminder to his crews of what they were dealing with. Quinlan had done the very first swab at St Mary's. A couple of weeks later, he was reading that sixteen people had died there. He remembers a dull shock coming over him. 'Oh my God' was the only reaction he could sum up. The staff in Mary's would look out of the windows and see a glimmer of light from the ambulance base. Testing was their only hope.

St Mary's would ask the ambulance staff in to do swabs at 10 or 11 p.m. 'We'd go over and do the swab and it would go into the lab with the rest of the items and come back and then you get the information maybe a day or two later that that person has passed away.' It hit the NAS staff hard. All too familiar with handling the aftermath of tragedies, this one was on their doorstep.

Fear for residents was real. 'Am I going to die?' some would ask staff, worried about the commotion and frightened calls from family members. Staff were terrified too, some staff members at times stepping out to the courtyard and weeping. 'The virus was there and it wasn't going to be stopped,' one member said. The barrage of daily news headlines about the hospital, the memo and the relentless demands were overwhelming.

A HSE webinar for staff managing nursing home outbreaks, which took place later in 2020, featured a contribution from Fiona Dunne, Assistant Director of Nursing at St Mary's. She told colleagues across the country that while the hospital and others like it prepared for a 'storm, it was a tsunami that was approaching'. Her presentation detailed the extraordinary challenges anyone who set foot in St Mary's in spring 2020 faced: 'Information overload ... isolating, traumatic, relentless for staff', the frequent change of guidance on PPE, a 'lack of understanding of the true reality of the situation ...' The list goes on.

Simone Comiskey, Director of Nursing, will remember the demands put upon her team, many of whom she'd worked alongside for years, and the strain for the rest of her life. Staff sickness took a relentless toll. Close contacts at that point were off work for sixteen days at a time, while many staff members became sick themselves. 'Over fifty per cent of our staff at one stage were out on sick leave,' Simone says. 'We had staff sick and then find out that staff that were sick had to go into hospital and then they were in intensive care. You just felt a huge amount of responsibility, you know?' Over a long career in nursing, Simone has seen it all. 'You work through a lot in nursing. You deal with outbreaks, you worked in ED, you work in intensive care. You have car crashes and what not but it was always *us* giving. Now the staff were affected as well, it was just huge.'

Staff members' family members were also affected. Some even had family members die from Covid-19. Despite bereavements, which left many feeling isolated in their darkest hour, they still turned out to work and continued caring. 'They were extremely challenging times,' says Aisling Coffey. 'The most complex and challenging times I think any of them have ever worked in.'

Extra staff were ferried in. Agency nurses were deployed from Wexford, and accommodated nearby. Healthcare assistants were drafted in. Others, working in activities like Catherine Lawlor, were deployed to the wards. The demands were never-ending but the staff kept showing up. 'We didn't know how bad it was going to get,' says Catherine, 'By God, it got bad.' Alison Fitzgerald says the dropping numbers of staff dialled up the fear factor. 'People were just thinking, "Is it going to be me next?" You were doing everything you could for it to not happen.'

So much of the focus for the staff in the middle of the disaster was on their residents. They were acutely aware that seeing staff members in full PPE was a disorienting and often frightening experience. 'You felt so sorry for the residents,' says Catherine, 'because they were used to the staff and then most of the staff were out sick … there was only one member of staff up there [on Tara Ward] apart from myself that the residents knew. You can imagine how they must have been so frightened – surrounded by strangers in gowns.'

Through layers of PPE, the single slightest recognition at times only highlighted the fear the residents must have faced regularly. 'All they can see is your eyes. Sometimes you'd hear them say "I know you", says Alison. 'Sometimes they'd recognize your voice.' New recruits and agency staff were brought into residents' rooms alongside staff who knew them, in an effort to reassure people, just to let them know they were safe.

As the month wore on, worried family members stood outside the hospital, often on window visits. Some struggled to see their loved one through the glare in the windows, adjusting their hand over their brows to try to make out a face, which was so close and yet had never seemed so far away. Having a family member living on the ground floor made things easier, according to families; other families, however, with relations on upper floors had to resort to standing on benches, tearfully calling out to their mother or father, maybe suffering from dementia, desperate to be understood or recognized from their position below. Information was hard to come by too. For family members, ringing the hospital was not a guaranteed source of answers or comfort. Families were often hearing about the situation for the first time in news coverage, a situation exacerbated by the staff shortages – there were just not enough people around to pick up the phone. Others were deeply upset by questions around funeral arrangements from staff members while their loved one was still battling for their life.

The social workers in St Mary's had to change all end-of-life plans during Covid. In normal circumstances, families would have extensive involvement in the lead-up to that time – they would be around the bed, they would have the chance to hold their loved ones and say their last goodbyes in the way they saw fit. Aisling Coffey and her team had to work on a contingency plan.

'Is there anything we could possibly do for your loved one at the end of their life?'

It was, to be frank, a 'terrible' situation, says Aisling, but the social workers were determined to do whatever they could. They asked residents and their families what comfort they wanted – whether there was a parish priest they wanted to contact or if there was music they wanted to be played. 'We tried to do anything we possibly could do,' says Aisling. 'So, we would have asked what kind and comforting words we'll whisper in the resident's ears and we went over and told them how much they were loved by their family and maybe their wife was waiting for them in heaven. Whatever the family felt was important.' Any personal belongings that could be brought close to the residents in those final moments were brought close. 'We were putting photos of wedding days, the squirrel teddy given by a grandchild, rosary beads, whatever it would be.'

Fr Pat Mernagh, the chaplain of the Defence Forces, based in McKee Barracks on Blackhorse Avenue just down from the Phoenix Park, was singled out for praise. He spoke to residents at length on the phone in their dying hours, reassuring them that loved ones who had gone before them would be waiting. His gentle manner was a gift in those hours when residents and staff alike needed a lift.

Alison Fitzgerald remembers the passing of one victim. The resident's family were present, separated from a final hug or a goodbye kiss on the forehead by the window. 'Her daughter just said to me, "Alison, I'm so glad you're here" because she was a resident who was previously upstairs and was transferred downstairs. I was so happy because they were a family that was in every day and to not be there at the end was devastating.' Having someone close at hand who knew the resident well was a comfort to the family. Fr Mernagh, despite the pressure and the trauma of the situation, was generous with his time, making sure to speak with the families at length about the lives their loved ones had led.

Aisling Coffey and the social workers were working eighteen-hour days, sometimes for twelve or thirteen days in a row, existing on pure adrenaline. This carried with it no small amount of trauma.

Frustrations grew with the media portrayal of what was happening. One senior nurse said that journalists or people on social media commented on St Mary's with 'no clue' what it was like to work there. 'It was awful, it was like a slap in the face,' she says, 'because staff were working so hard. And you've these bastards out there who have no idea what it's like to work ...' She stops herself finishing the sentence.

Alison Fitzgerald agrees. Trudging in from a day working in torturous heat in boiler suit-level PPE, looking after frightened residents, trying to get through every hour as it came, she met her husband in the kitchen. He was reading an article about the deaths in St Mary's and asked her about it. 'Friends of mine would say, "Oh God, Alison, I read that article," and I said, "Listen, it is nothing like that."' She told her husband and friends that 'Everybody in the hospital, everyone, was doing their utter best. We did everything we could.'

In previous years, when someone who lived in St Mary's died, the staff would mark it. They would line the courtyard in a guard of honour, waiting to say goodbye to a member of the St Mary's family. 'In some cases we would walk all the way over to the gate,' says Alison, 'because that is the very, very last thing we can do for them and their family.' This was another important custom broken by the virus. 'They were taken out a side door,' says Alison. 'Thank God families weren't there to see that because that was so distressing.'

There was no opportunity for families to say a peaceful and dignified goodbye in person to their loved one, there was no time to reflect as their loved one was laid out, no time to see them in a coffin, there was no time for any of these parting moments, replaced as they were with Covid protocols. Staff worry about how this compounded grief and what carrying this loss will mean for them in years to come. 'It is a huge loss when so many people are sick and passing away very close together. It was devastating for staff as well. I can't imagine what pain the families were going through. They were going through an awful lot of pain,' says Alison.

Residents themselves were losing friends they had lived with for years to the virus.

In some cases, people didn't know for quite some time that the person in the room next door had died. Clippings and cut-outs from the *Irish Independent* or RIP.ie were given to residents in St Mary's who had lost friends and neighbours they'd spent so many happy times with – at bingo, at dinner, at gardening club. The fear that must have been felt by those in their final months in Covid-driven isolation is difficult to face or comprehend. They lost friends, they lost their community. Their loved ones were kept away as their time on earth drew to an end.

Rosie Hegarty, in her room in St Mary's, knew the virus was getting closer. At the beginning of April, the first case on her ward was confirmed. She was aware that residents elsewhere in the hospital had died. Her niece Jane Carrigan says that Rosie was very clear that if she got Covid it would be the end for her. In a conversation with her nephew Bernard, she stoically told him she believed she would die if the virus did breach St Mary's. She had poor kidney function and was very aware of how damaging even a bad cold could be for her quality of life at this point. Her mind was as sharp as a tack, her body was vulnerable.

On 19 April 2020, Rosie Hegarty had a cough. The staff kept the family informed, but the family was keen to hear from Rosie herself. After a few missed calls, fraught with worry, Jane got hold of her. Rosie said she'd been given a bit of oxygen and was feeling better for it and was now happily having her

141

dinner. 'I'll give Cathy a ring later on,' she said, conscious that her nieces were worried about her.

The call didn't come. 'We knew at that stage,' says Jane – Rosie was in trouble. It had been reported just days earlier that eleven deaths had been confirmed by St Mary's, with ten of those residents Covid positive. Rosie would have been aware of all of this, Jane says. 'You're looking at a catastrophe happening around you but you only really feel like you're a bit player.'

An article in that weekend's *Sunday Independent* by journalist Ciara Dwyer spoke about her own experiences of St Mary's and those of her mother, a resident there. She praised the staff and the lengths to which they went to protect her mum and to get good information to the family in the middle of a tempest. The article was accompanied by a photograph of Ciara standing on the grounds outside St Mary's, waving up at her mother who was above on a second-floor balcony, accompanied by staff clad in heavy PPE. This was the first time some families became aware of the possibility of window visits.

Jane and Cathy immediately seized on this and were out the very next day. On that day, Monday the twentieth, Rosie was due to be tested; serial testing was being implemented throughout the hospital to try to map the scale of the outbreak across St Mary's. The family hoped against hope that Rosie's test wouldn't reveal Covid. The following day, on another window visit, they happened across a young doctor, who they saw again on visits over the days ahead.

He came out to the Carrigans and said, 'I'm sorry. I'm sorry I'm telling you this here.' He explained that a decision might have to be made about ventilation later. Jane, Cathy and Rosie's family were aware of Rosie's own wishes – 'she didn't want medical intervention'. The doctor himself was kind, as Jane remembers so many staff were through the darkest days. He told her, she says, 'We don't know what to do to treat people, we're just giving oxygen. Sometimes people seem to recover quickly, and then if they don't recover then we know they're not going to recover, but that's just what I'm seeing.' The honesty was appreciated. It was a way of understanding the terrible situation. Rosie herself was in and out of consciousness, in a state of semi-sleep.

After her positive test, the staff at St Mary's would call Cathy almost on the dot at 8.50 every morning: 'She's comfortable, she had a good night's sleep.' The family allowed themselves to hope. 'When someone rings you and says someone you love has had a good night … suddenly "Oh wow, that's a great night! That's three good nights in a row, brilliant."'

One morning, 8.50 came and 8.50 passed without a call. 'That's when we knew.'

On Monday 27 April, Rosie died.

Cathy was called at 9.30 that morning to tell her that Rosie had passed. The family went to the window. They didn't expect to see her but felt they should mark Rosie's passing. As chance would have it, one of the nurses heard them from inside the room and lifted up the curtain so they could see Rosie. 'It was really lovely to see, she looked peaceful and we could see how she was dressed.' It was some comfort to the family but they were angry underneath it all. They felt bereft they couldn't be there for Rosie's final moments or say goodbye to her.

Jane wrote to the *Irish Times* that day. She wanted to make sure the public knew what it was like for the residents of nursing homes in their final days, 'to say something about how she lived and how she died.' Jane wrote with pain. 'There was an awful injustice done because she had been taking as many precautions as I had and more. I couldn't understand how this could happen.' The letter read:

Sir, – From her private bedroom in St Mary's Hospital, Phoenix Park, my aunt watched the news and read the papers.

At the beginning of March, she decided to stop going to dinner in the communal dining room and instead had food brought to her room. She kept a hand sanitiser by her bed.

She listened to Leo Varadkar's announcement on March 12th.

On March 17th, she waved at family members through her ground-floor window for the last time. Restricted physical mobility was not new to her and the phone and the post became her communication with the outside world.

On March 29th, the nursing home rang us to tell us there was a case of Covid-19 in the facility.

The next day, she rang to let us know that fact too.

On April 19th, my aunt began displaying symptoms.

On April 25th, we learned her test result came back positive.

My wonderful aunt, Mrs Rose Hegarty, died on April 27th, 2020.

Each sentence tells a story. I hope we get to hear the full one. – Yours, etc,
JANE CARRIGAN,
Dublin 11.

Jane's family are one of many calling for a full inquiry into St Mary's and all the nursing homes that suffered in the pandemic. 'I think Leo Varadkar said something in his speech [St Patrick's Day, 2020] about how "when things were at their worst, we were at our best". I don't think we were at our best. Some things we did well and others we didn't. I think our most vulnerable cohort were actually in nursing homes that are almost hidden away in some respects.' The families calling for an inquiry are a group, spread across the country, left bereft. They suffer the loss of a loved one without closure, years before their time, without the chance to whisper 'I love you' one last time. Theirs was a stolen goodbye.

Twenty-four residents died in the outbreak in St Mary's Hospital across the month of April. It was a devastating loss of life, one keenly felt by all who were associated with the nursing home.

In writing this chapter about the experiences of those who lived through the times of St Mary's, interviews with staff members Director of Nursing Simone Comiskey; Essene Cassidy, Head of Service – Older Persons for CHO Dublin North City and County (DNCC); Director of Nursing for DNCC's Community Units Caroline Gourley; and St Mary's Principal Social Worker Aisling Coffey, were held simultaneously at St Mary's.

As the interviews wrapped up, Caroline Gourley and Aisling Coffey's contrasting views on how to cope with what was lived through in those dark days were revelatory.

Caroline says her strongest memory will be one of the resilience and kindness, the incredible efforts of residents, families and staff who were put through an experience none of them could ever have expected or would ever have wished upon anyone.

Aisling's memory? 'I'm sorry to say, but for me, it'll be the loss. It will be. I don't think that'll ever leave any of us. Just who we'd lost and the characters we've lost. It's a great sadness to carry around but I don't see it leaving us any time soon nor leaving others that are affected either … You see the kindness in people, the humanity, the decency, but there is still the sorrow. I don't think that sorrow is going to lift any time soon. It can't. It's too deep.'

Caroline agreed that the sense of loss was 'very deep' but stressed that 'you have to see the other side of it' or 'the silver lining', she says. 'If you actually focus on the loss all the time, it will destroy you.'

The competing sides of grief and coping, the contrasting pain of loss and the hope borne of resilience are ones widely felt by those who worked in health and residential care throughout the pandemic.

Caroline Gourley says that if she focused on the loss as Aisling does, she 'would probably end up rocking in a corner' with a bottle of whiskey. 'If I concentrate on that and if I put that to the fore, I couldn't, it would consume me.'

For Aisling Coffey, it's a different view. 'I understand that, Caroline,' she said, 'but when I think about it I cry. I nearly cry every day thinking about it because it's still … it's a very deep wound. I completely understand what you're saying, I think we're all coping in different ways.' It's a point they agree on. Everyone who has gone through a traumatic experience like this, stretched out across weeks or months of turmoil and loss, will carry it with them. How they process it is something that will be individual to each of them; neither way is the wrong one.

At the time of writing, an independent investigation into the protected disclosure by a member of staff into PPE, the preparations for and the response to Covid-19 in St Mary's was a year into its work. Several families of residents have come forward to corroborate the claims within and are still searching for answers.

Chapter 10: The New Normal

The Fine Gael-led caretaker administration was enjoying a revival in its political fortunes. At the end of March, opinion pollsters Red C had Leo Varadkar's party on thirty-four per cent, up a massive thirteen per cent. Sinn Féin were second on twenty-eight per cent. Fianna Fáil were down on eighteen per cent. After an abysmal result for Fine Gael in the general election, last in a three-horse race, the turnabout was Lazarene. And the world took notice. The *New York Times* wrote about how the pandemic 'rescued the political image of Ireland's leader', who won praise for re-registering as a doctor to take phone calls for Covid assessments, while comparisons were immediately drawn with the deepening tragedy in Britain under Boris Johnson.

Minister Shane Ross, in the final leg of his run in government, outlined in his book *In Bed with the Blueshirts* how he suspected the emergency 'was being milked for all it was worth' by Fine Gael's ministers and spin doctors. 'Democracy took a rest for four months.'

Suspicions were not new to Ross, who was one of many to grapple with the tumult of video-link Cabinet meetings. Briefings were organized with the CMO and senior civil servants like Martin Fraser and Brian Murphy to give ministers, left out of the big meetings of the sub-committee, the chance to engage with the public health advisers face to face and see what they were made of.

147

Ministers like Michael Ring, Eoghan Murphy and Michael Creed were the most vocal critics of the strict adherence to the dogma of public health. At one briefing, via video link, sitting at home in Westport in front of newspaper cut-outs of election triumphs past, a tired-looking Ring let rip at Tony Holohan. He accused the CMO of locking people up 'in a police state' and claimed that people would soon be 'on the streets' in uprising against the lockdown.

It was around this time that some members of the Cabinet lost their 'awe' of the CMO. There was a growing sense of grievance among some ministers, with suspicions that Holohan's role was overshadowing their own. The emergence of Holohan as a 'father of the nation' or heroic figure was uncomfortable for ministers, who sought to clip his wings, some privately assessing that his ability to influence the populace and politicians had marked him out as the 'most powerful figure in the history of Irish public life'.

Martin Fraser was among those who was known to have misgivings about Holohan's role, some ministers suggesting his nose was put out of joint by the fact that a civil servant at least two rungs down from Fraser had become a seemingly untouchable figure. Fraser had Holohan's back, though, marshalling the sceptics and reading them the riot act. The message was clear – a misstep now, even as the days grew brighter and the longing for summer more palpable, could be catastrophic.

Fraser's role had grown, too. After almost a decade as the civil service's most senior figure, and many years of high-level service before that under the Cowen and Ahern governments, ministers could clearly see his hand in political matters. 'He understands politics. He's not partisan but very political.' That expertise would come to the fore quite regularly at Cabinet. Varadkar as Taoiseach would go around the Cabinet table or across his ministers linking in via video, and ask

Martin Fraser's opinion alongside the actual members of the Government.

Meetings between Varadkar and his advisors, and Fraser and his officials, would often see this prowess come to the fore, with Fraser overriding all other advisers offering political advice to the Taoiseach. 'He was working his power very effectively indeed,' says one minister, who described Fraser as having a network in the 'undergrowth' of the civil service while also knowing everything going on at Cabinet. 'He's incredibly strong – clever and informed. He's almost unchallengeable.'

For a figure so influential and well connected, Fraser has little public persona. The Malahide man would frequently be seen arriving into Government Buildings in his Dublin GAA bobble hat and a hulking pair of Beats headphones. If that didn't betray his out-of-work passions, his official diaries over recent years do, laden as they are with markers of reminders to get to a television for Super Bowls and Liverpool matches and notes for concerts like Regina Spektor, The National and Jay-Z.

The reliance on internet connections led to shaky virtual Cabinet sessions. Ross was suspicious that his microphone was being deliberately muted at times by Fine Gael, a worry that no doubt has crossed the minds of many business people in remote meetings through 2020 and 2021.

As the Government began manoeuvres to reopen the country, the behavioural scientists of the Economic and Social Research Institute (ESRI) were consulted for their expertise. Professor Pete Lunn and his colleagues had been monitoring public attitudes. 'People were really worried,' he says, 'that as soon as you open the gate a little bit people come flooding out. They were also worried, however, about mental health and wellbeing. That side was looking really ugly.' The ESRI gauged that people wanted hope, optimism and something to look forward to.

In April, it 'road-tested' an experiment of how people would react to certain announcements of strategies for exiting the first lockdown. It was designed to look like a government announcement. It suggested that restrictions would be eased from 5 May and reviewed again in June, with measures like the 2km limit relaxed and people over the age of seventy allowed to leave homes for 'safe walks' for up to thirty minutes per day.

Someone taking part in the study took a photo of it and stuck it online.

A message came through from one of Lunn's team – 'Jesus Christ, our experiment is on Twitter.' Panic ensued. 'We were doing this quietly ahead of the first restrictions lifting and it was very sensitive stuff.' Lunn called the Department of Health and held his hands up. 'I'm very sorry about this, I thought you should know.'

It was too late. The Department's press office and Government Buildings were already fielding calls. The press office 'had no idea that this was funded research and was actually something they'd commissioned. So, totally understandably, they dismissed it but the journalists then swallowed it was fake.'

The leak caused jitters in the ESRI, which was clear that whatever the strategy, it was important for the public to think, 'Yes, that makes sense. I can sign up to that.' With isolation and wellbeing taking a hit across the country, getting the messaging right was essential.

* * * *

Finbarr O'Sullivan was fourteen years in An Post in Douglas, outside Cork city. In those fourteen years, he'd done everything – foot soldier, driving a truck, working nights sorting mail – but most of all delivering post. None of his fourteen years of service could compare to this. With older people isolating at home, families working from their own houses and people relying more than ever on deliveries and letters to stay connected, the role of delivery services grew ever more important in people's lives.

It was off-the-wall busy. 'It was so hectic I had to half the delivery and see them every second day,' he says; 'half a normal delivery route ended up being a day and a half's work.' There were parcels on top of parcels on top of parcels. Two hundred of them every single day. He obsessed about the workload. His fiancée recalls hearing him talking about boxes in his sleep.

Throughout March and April, people would come to the door or to the front wall to chat with him, or vent, craving human contact. 'I was very aware that we were the only people that some would see in a day.' He'd worry about them and what was going on behind closed doors. These were customers and members of his community he'd see every day. He'd knock on doors to check that everything was okay.

The pressure was severe but everyone was aware of the increased demands of the job. At times, post workers were out seven days a week, and they became a lifeline of connection in a time that had shrunk people's world to the end of their garden path.

'I felt like a somebody, not just "your man there with the box." It was great to be valued and needed and being needed would give you a big head!' Finbarr jokes. 'We were pillars of the community again.'

Community outreach workers and volunteers played a huge role too in keeping people in lockdown connected. Former Mayo GAA star David Brady and League of Ireland footballer Conan Byrne organized ex-players and officials from the world of sport to ring older people or those who were isolating for some company and an opportunity to chat about past glories or the chances that had passed Mayo by. It was an enormous success. People in their eighties and nineties opening up about their loneliness and whether someone would drop the shopping in to them the next day; people weeping about missing their grandchildren or about friends or loved ones who had passed. Sport was only the key to open the door to deeper conversation. Dozens volunteered to make and take the calls. The work of volunteers like David and Conan and of others operating off their own bat in the community, delivering care parcels or food to cocooning neighbours was the centre of much-deserved attention in the early pandemic, and worthy of remembering in the darker days to come.

Another group of unsung heroes were those at the frontline of social protection. Within the first two weeks of the Pandemic Unemployment Payment, or PUP, being introduced, welfare staff processed almost 400,000 applications from people who had been laid off. It was equivalent to handling nineteen months' worth of claims in the space of a single fortnight. Before the PUP was announced in March, Finance Minister Paschal Donohoe was in his office when there was a knock on the door. A leading official came in bearing bad news on a scale beyond comprehension to the minder of the State's coffers. 'We think we could have six hundred thousand people unemployed within the next week,' the official said. 'As good as the systems are ... they're not going to process applications for that many people. We can't do it.'

PUP and the Employment Wage Subsidy Scheme (EWSS) were crafted over a weekend between Donohoe, DPER Secretary General Robert Watt, Niall Cody of the Revenue Commissioners and other officials from the Department of Employment Affairs and Social Protection. Donohoe maintains that the only intervention bigger than the PUP and EWSS in the history of the State was the bank guarantee of 2008.

Intreo offices around the country had to shut after the first wave of restrictions saw 80,000 people forced to queue outside at a time when the Government was pleading with people not to gather together. Everything went online in a matter of days, and in an instant, sixty per cent of welfare officers were working from their spare rooms and home offices.

They worked exceptionally long hours, right through the night in many cases, over kitchen tables and 2 a.m. cups of coffee, 'terrified that people wouldn't get their payments'. One Intreo worker who spoke on condition of anonymity said she had 'nightmares' about the workload. It was like the economic crash of 2011, but overnight and multiplied.

It wasn't plain sailing, and rows between Social Protection and Public Expenditure did happen – as they had over the years. In one Budget meeting before the pandemic, the DPER Secretary General is understood to have banged the table in frustration and told officials, including Minister Regina Doherty, that her Department was running the risk of becoming the new Department of Health.

The mindset of careful purse-management had to change. Many ministers and their officials tried to force the issue, pointing the finger at DPER for being too careful about the State's money at a time when it was being modelled that as many as 50,000 were at risk of dying. 'You were going "Are you off your rocker?" at some of the economic hawks,' says one member of the Cabinet. If the payments were cut, and there was a chance they might be, the Government feared a complete breakdown in social cohesion.

* * * *

The lockdown persisted as the first wave continued. On 10 April, Varadkar announced that due to the ongoing uncertainty the restrictions would continue until 5 May at the earliest. When that decision was made, there was shock.

Holohan arrived in the canteen at the Department of Health, where Harris was chatting with an adviser. 'Look,' Holohan said,

'I'll brief you properly when we're finished here but … just to say, no change until …' The adviser collapsed in tears. 'I just started bawling my eyes out. Tony was just standing there going "What?" It was just a moment where it hit me all at once. This isn't going to be a short-term thing.'

It was a dawning realization that hit many people in April. The early lockdown's sense of unity, of novelty, was ebbing away. Banana bread baking and sourdough starters, home fitness programmes and *Normal People* would soon give way to crippling ennui. A realization that 'the new normal' was anything but.

As the growth rate of cases tapered off, deaths continued to rise. Day after day in mid-April, 'forty-four new deaths reported … forty-one new deaths reported … thirty-nine … seventy-seven new deaths reported.' By the end of the month, the confirmed death toll had passed one thousand.

On 21 April, Dr Tony Holohan told a press conference that the curve had been flattened. With summer on the horizon, the clamour began for a roadmap out of restrictions. The ESRI was wargaming how the announcement would be received by the public. NPHET was focusing on urging people to stay the course and thanking them for their work in staving off a devastating peak that would have overwhelmed the country's hospitals.

The reopening roadmap began across three phases. Phase One on 18 May saw the 2km limit pushed out to 5km, construction workers returning to sites across the country, outdoor activities and locations like popular beaches and national parks reopening and shops like hardware stores – though not homeware stores – reopening for business.

On 8 June, it was Phase Two Plus with people over seventy finally allowed to welcome others into their homes; travel limits extended to county boundaries or within 20km of home; funeral attendances expanded to twenty-five people;

and people being urged to 'stay local' rather than to 'stay at home'.

The final phase, Phase Three, was announced on the final day of the caretaker government on 25 June. Ongoing talks with Fianna Fáil and the Greens had borne fruit. The suspicion among political circles was that Leo Varadkar had announced the roadmap before the new Government could come into play. 'There was probably a reluctance to leave it for the new Government,' says one Fine Gael minister. The caretaker administration was over. Housing Minister Eoghan Murphy smoked a cigarette in the courtyard with Minister for Disability Issues Finian McGrath. Other ministers, riding off into the sunset, slung their jackets over their shoulders. The Independent Alliance posed for photos, Shane Ross beaming for the cameras.

Varadkar, job completed, stepped out into the courtyard at Dublin Castle on 25 June with his party riding high in the polls. He felt unburdened and at the top of his game. The Taoiseach's habit of bringing pop culture references into his speeches had continued. He had quoted variously from *Terminator 2*, *The Lord of the Rings*, singer-songwriter Dermot Kennedy and even teen comedy *Mean Girls*, following a bet with actor Sean Astin facilitated on RTÉ Radio. There would be no quote that evening. 'None are needed,' he told the nation. 'Until now we needed some hope to cling to, but your actions have turned that hope into a reality.'

Some in government, particularly those in the Independent Alliance, who were on the way out, found the references immature and childish. Varadkar defends them, saying that far too much was read into their use. 'I was a little bit more willing just to be myself and maybe take a few little risks and throw in quotes. I mightn't have done the *Mean Girls* one again if I could go back. The other ones I thought were reasonable,' he says.

What followed was one of the strangest encounters I had

in the early pandemic. Varadkar caught sight of the Virgin Media News camera and myself standing at the corner of the courtyard and made a beeline for us.

'Hey neighbour!' he called, as his aide and Garda drivers waited for him beside the car. I thought I misheard him. Camera operator Joan McKenna had focused her lens on what had been the departing Taoiseach, thinking there'd be a tracking shot of his car leaving for the last time. As he turned to walk towards the camera, we thought he might be coming to give us a quick parting comment.

'Hey neighbour!' Varadkar called again as he came closer. The pictures were being broadcast live picture-in-picture in a split screen with a colleague's live report. A cold flush came over me, fearing the sound was being broadcast in anticipation of an unprompted Varadkar interview.

It was clear the Taoiseach had learned that I was living in a house-share in his home patch of Castleknock. 'When are we going for a pint?,' he said as he walked straight up to me. 'We're live, Taoiseach,' I muttered.

'Sorry?' he asked.

I'm not one for going for drinks with politicians, and the idea of the suggestion being aired publicly was not one I particularly fancied.

'Our picture is live,' I said, before asking if he was giving us an interview. At that point he said, 'Oh, no' and quickly turned on his heel.

In my earpiece, I heard our director ask: 'What was that? Was he going to give you an interview?'

I was mortified. Fortunately, our sound wasn't being aired live, but studio was seconds from doing so. My phone vibrated into life – several texts were asking what Varadkar said to me. Now they know. That's how close Leo Varadkar's final televised words to the public as Taoiseach were to being 'Are we going for a pint?'

Some in health circles and in government have compared Varadkar's speech that day to the George W. Bush 'Mission Accomplished' announcement on the deck of an aircraft carrier in March 2003, years before the war in Iraq had ended.

'He was trying to create a sense of "I've sorted it"; says one public health doctor who says that Varadkar was handing it over to the next Taoiseach with a sense of 'Don't fuck it up now'. Others at the Cabinet table and in health officialdom believe he was speaking to a much-improved situation. 'The mission *was* accomplished at the time,' says one minister. 'It was time for the country to open up.'

Varadkar himself denies that was the idea. 'That wasn't the message,' he says. 'I was always aware that, like the 1918 pandemic, there could be a second wave and had said so publicly. That was always a possibility. I probably didn't say that in the speech but I certainly would have said before that "this hasn't gone away, you know". I think I said I thought another national lockdown was unlikely and I did think that.'

The wartime caretaker government had ended its term in office and even if the ministers of Fine Gael were over it, the pandemic was not over.

PART II

Chapter 11: The Changeover

Micheál Martin had to be Taoiseach. There were no two ways about it. Either he got the job first or he was finished.

Fianna Fáil were, to start with, the only enthusiastic participants in the three-legged stool of the new coalition, with Martin in the driver's seat and Varadkar happy to give way. The decisions around portfolios would be key to the balancing act of former foes and sworn enemies. It was, as the historian Doris Kearns Goodwin described Abraham Lincoln's war cabinet, a *Team of Rivals*.

Fine Gael were hammered on health and housing during the election. Those departments would need to switch hands. This left Simon Harris on the outside. Harris, who for all the world knew politically that getting out of the most difficult, most sprawling, most unforgiving department of all to navigate would be good for his future career. But he wanted more. Between packing his boxes back in February and actually having to leave in June, he had formed a bond with officials and staff in the Department fighting in the trenches on those long, dark nights in the early spring. He admits he was 'gutted' on a personal level, having built those links. 'I felt the job wasn't fully done,' he says. 'I was talking to the people of Ireland almost constantly on TV or radio or social media. You don't like leaving your team mid-battle.'

Close colleagues say he wanted to keep the job. In fact, he

161

raised the idea of staying on for a few months with the outgoing Taoiseach Leo Varadkar. If there was any chance, he said, of keeping going in the portfolio while the pandemic continued, he really would like to. He held out hope. The links he built with Micheál Martin gave him reason to feel perhaps he could stay on.

In private conversations his confidantes told officials he would go back in the morning if he was offered the gig. Most of them thought he was mad to even think about it.

Speculation turned to who would now occupy the minister's office at the Department of Health. In the corridors and car parks of Leinster House, whispers mentioned Fianna Fáil stalwarts:

'Dara Calleary? He'd be good. He gets it.'

'Barry Cowen? He'll need a seat at the table.'

'What about Michael McGrath? He's big into the Covid stuff. He has the head for Health.'

Leo Varadkar reckoned it might be Calleary or Cowen. Whispers around Miesian Plaza suggested that Michael McGrath would be a heavyweight appointment to the job. In the end, few predicted that Fianna Fáil's Health Spokesperson Stephen Donnelly would be the man for the job.

The appointment of the Wicklow TD shouldn't have been much of a surprise, and yet it was. Fianna Fáil insiders were outraged. 'One of the things that pisses Fianna Fáil off is that it's not as though we're a talent-free zone,' in the words of one senior TD. 'Micheál went out of his way to pick a guy who is only in the party about two years and who had described Fianna Fáil as being a cowboy outfit. He started his career in the 2011 election by hammering us as being incompetent and inept. That affects people's thinking and Jesus, we just felt Micheál should have picked someone from Fianna Fáil who was there a while who had been through all the battles.'

Donnelly and Harris have been rivals at constituency and national level for years. While there has rarely been any face-to-face animosity between the pair since the formation of the Government, there have been suspicions of briefing and counter-briefing by proxies and loyal colleagues. It's been a distraction at times, colleagues at Cabinet say.

The Greens in particular would take issue with leaking and briefing against members of the Government from inside the tent. 'If you want to be leader of your party, and you get the reputation of being someone who is a bit "not to be trusted", in the long run is that going to be a clever strategy?' asks Eamon Ryan. 'I don't think so. If you are slightly undermining your own reputation, that will come back to haunt you.'

Simon Harris had left a letter on the minister's desk on his way out the door, not knowing who his successor would be. It wished them well, saying that they would be well served by the people in the Department, who were exhausted and had worked themselves to the bone during the first wave. The job would be lonely and toilsome, but the office had an ability to make a profound impact on people's lives. There was no reply to the letter, no acknowledgement of its receipt. Neither was there any handover. Department staffers felt a catch-up between Harris and Donnelly would have been helpful given the demands of the position, the unique situation and the spotlight Health was under.

As Ireland was marking its departure from the first phase of the pandemic, Dr Tony Holohan was making way for personal reasons. His wife, Dr Emer Holohan, was diagnosed with multiple myeloma, a blood cancer, in 2012. After a number of difficult years of illness, Emer was admitted to palliative care at the end of June. At an early meeting with the new minister, Holohan told him that he wasn't going to be around for long. It was time to go home.

News of Holohan's departure hit close colleagues hard. Officials, his clerical staff, the Communications team and others across the building, had felt guided by Holohan through the uncertainty of the first wave. In a pre-press conference meeting, word got out that something was up. Holohan drafted his remarks. They were checked and double-checked. Officials increased the font size to enable the CMO to read the statement without his glasses. It was an overwhelmingly emotional moment for those who worked on the communications.

The news hadn't reached the journalists in the press room. It was a Friday evening. The situation across the country was improving. The 'draw' of the NPHET press briefings was fading. A press photographer stepped out through the glass doors of the briefing room mere minutes into the latest briefing. Deirdre Watters, the Head of Communications, whispered to him that he'd want to come back for the end of it.

'I have a personal statement I'm going to read, if that's okay,' Holohan said. 'From today, I will be taking time out from all of my work commitments to be with my family. I now want to give my energy, attention and all of my time to Emer and to our two teenage children, Clodagh and Ronan. As a husband and father, and as a public health doctor, I'm conscious that we all have been through tough times together over the last number of months and many families across the country have been affected by the course of Covid-19, suffering pain and loss of loved ones.'

Holohan was flanked by Professor Philip Nolan to his right and Dr Ronan Glynn to his left. Nolan had known Tony and Emer for decades, going back to college, when they graduated together at UCD. They had interned together but didn't have a huge amount of contact until Holohan called Nolan at eight o'clock one Saturday morning in March to tell him his services were needed. 'We're using some modelling information that we've got from the United Kingdom, but we can't just keep looking at their copybook. We'll have to do some homework of our own,' he told him.

Ronan Glynn was appointed Acting CMO in Holohan's stead.

Holohan and Glynn had a bond dating back to before the pandemic. Emer had put him on Tony's radar, having worked with Ronan in public health medicine. Five years previous, Glynn came to the CMO's office on a six-month attachment. 'Oh yeah,' Emer had commented to Tony, 'you're getting this Ronan Glynn guy coming in? I have to say, he's really good.'

Holohan says, smiling, 'I can still remember coming out of my office in Hawkins House, the old Department building, and I had an anteroom outside my office. There was Ronan Glynn, sitting in the chair in the anteroom. He's only a slip of a fella, you know. I liked him from the off. I really did.' Glynn quickly became Holohan's right-hand man. The man referred to as 'the apprentice' would now be stepping into the breach to command NPHET's response.

Tributes to Holohan rolled in. From the Taoiseach, from Simon Harris, from Stephen Donnelly, from across political and civic life. Things would now be very different.

* * * *

In mere days, the State's entire leadership base for the pandemic had changed. The Taoiseach was rotated. The Health Minister had changed. The Chief Medical Officer was on leave of absence. The Department of Health's top civil servant, Secretary General Jim Breslin, was also out, following Simon Harris to the new Department of Further Education.

That Donnelly was left in charge of the Department without a secretary general or long-standing CMO is now seen as a major blunder by the incoming Government. Some in Fianna Fáil have privately come back to it as something that could have protected Donnelly from the pitfalls of the hard months of media coverage that followed. Without it, he was left handling the running of the Department with few allies. 'He was thrown in at the deep end,' says one Health source, 'and it was sink or swim.'

165

Dr Colm O'Reardon was appointed interim Secretary General and was well liked across the civil service and in the Department, but a temporary secretary general had no real power.

Micheál Martin became frustrated. New regulations from Health were lagging behind. He urged Martin Fraser, now serving under his third Taoiseach, to get a competition going to add real firepower to the top of the Department of Health again and offer assistance to Donnelly in a department the Taoiseach knew only too well could swallow you whole.

There would be tougher moments ahead. Just seventeen days into the new Government, Martin sacked Agriculture Minister Barry Cowen. Cowen had refused to address the Dáil in relation to the controversy over a drink-driving ban he had received four years earlier. Micheál Martin's coalition leaders agreed with the decision to end what Martin described as 'damaging to the ongoing work of government'.

For Martin, losing one Minister for Agriculture was a blow, but one that could be overcome. The loss of another in quick succession was what Socialist TD Mick Barry would describe as an 'omnishambles', and People Before Profit's Paul Murphy would call a 'dumpster fire'.

* * * *

Aoife Grace Moore didn't even know there was an Oireachtas Golf Society. Less than a year into their jobs as political correspondents with the *Irish Examiner*, Moore and her colleague Paul Hosford were still getting to grips with their new roles and trying to build a familiarity with the colourful personalities and groupings around the Dáil.

The story of their lives landed in their lap. An anonymous email popped into the *Examiner* inbox. The attachment was a video of a floorpan of multiple tables for guests at an Oireachtas

Golf Society dinner at the Station House Hotel in Clifden. 'Surely not,' they reasoned with each other, as the loop of names – a cabinet minister, senators, an EU Commissioner and a Supreme Court judge – slowly crawled across their phone screens. A gathering of that size broke the Government's own restrictions.

Moore rang the hotel, asking casually whether or not the dinner had gone ahead the night before. It had. Eighty people had been there. They were on. They divvied up the names, scoured around for phone numbers and began the task of working out who had been there and who hadn't.

Dara Calleary, the Mayo TD and new Minister for Agriculture, was the first to get a call from Aoife Moore. He instantly knew the jig was up. 'It was a very, very stupid thing to have done,' says Calleary, looking back. 'I did it with the best of intentions.' He had attended the event to honour Mark Killilea, one of his mentors.

If the two journalists didn't know they had something major on their hands, the fact that attendees started 'lying' to Moore only encouraged them. Some attendees said that everyone attending was in one room. Others said two rooms. One told Hosford there were multiple rooms. The two journalists felt their numbers were being passed around once those who were there sussed that something was up. People stopped answering calls, the easiest way to avoid being swiftly dragged into a whirlpool just beginning to stir.

'I phoned numerous other people, all men,' says Moore, 'because there was only one woman there of her own volition. There was no other woman there who wasn't a partner of someone else.'

They had to work quickly. Someone else had the story. Calleary's special adviser was working on a statement to issue to the *Examiner* and let Moore know that another publication had been in touch. The story was leaking. Acting CMO

Dr Ronan Glynn was hosting the NPHET press briefing that evening and was on the receiving end of some coded, and carefully worded, questions from journalists who had been tipped off that something was brewing.

The *Examiner* raced to get the story past the lawyers and published online. Moore tweeted the link as soon as Hosford had it over to her. 'Go, go, go.' It instantly made waves. The two journalists' phones exploded with messages and calls from people who were personally anguished by the breaking of the rules.

As soon as the story splashed, Calleary's inbox was overloaded too. People told the minister how they couldn't go to funerals, they couldn't see their families, they weren't in the room with their loved ones when they died in hospital. He felt each and every one of them as he scrolled through them. Calleary realized that he had to go. 'It wouldn't be right for me not to resign,' he said. 'I don't try to cause insult. I don't try to cause hurt to people in my way of doing politics. I certainly did feel that.'

Calleary was gone the next morning. A number of Fine Gael senators who had been at the dinner were forced to resign the party whip. After days of controversy and initial stubborn refusal to go, EU Commissioner Phil Hogan stood down from his post. Séamus Woulfe, the former Attorney General and recently appointed Supreme Court judge, stayed on under huge external pressure.

RTÉ's *Liveline* with Joe Duffy was inundated with upset callers. It was the cry of an exhausted and angry nation. 'It's one rule for them and another for the rest of us' was the prevailing emotion. Some are more equal than others.

Moore, heading to Newry to pick up her wedding dress, stopped twice to take radio interviews about what was quickly becoming known as Golfgate. Her political editor, Daniel McConnell, asked her to draft a column for Saturday's front

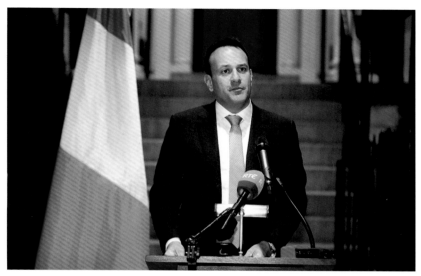

'I need to speak to you about the coronavirus.' An exhausted Leo Varadkar arrives at the podium to announce the first Covid-19 restrictions from Blair House, Washington DC. (*PA Images / Alamy Photo*)

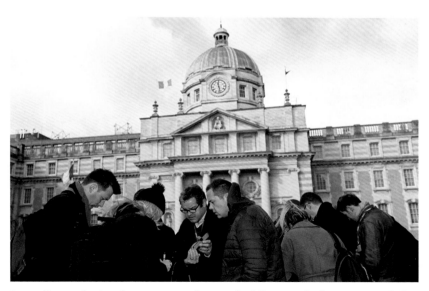

Journalists, gathering for a news conference, huddle around phones to watch Leo Varadkar's address from Washington ahead of the imposition of the first restrictions in Ireland. (*PA Images / Alamy Photo*)

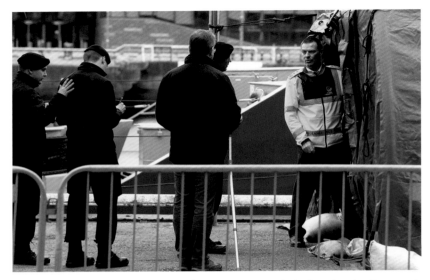

All hands on deck: the crew of the LÉ Samuel Beckett docked at Sir John Rogerson's Quay to run a swabbing centre. Its 'soft launch' would be the only queue in Dublin on St Patrick's Day. Richard Quinlan of the National Ambulance Service directs traffic. (*PA Images / Alamy Photo*)

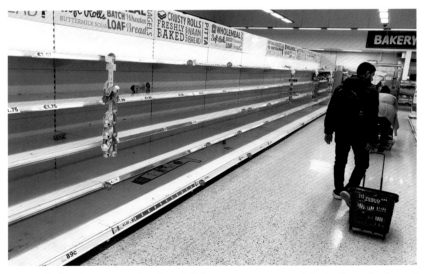

Empty shelves in supermarket bread aisles were a common sight in the early days of lockdown. (*PA Images / Alamy Photo*)

21 March, 2020: Mícheál Ó Gallachóir shows off his newborn son Faolán to his father Michael. The meeting of three generations, separated by window glass, would go viral as a symbol of lockdown separations. (*Mícheál Ó Gallachóir*)

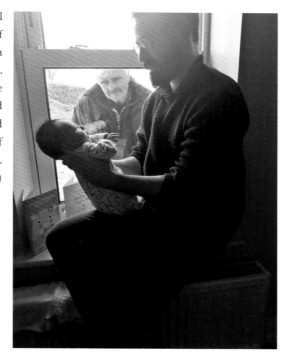

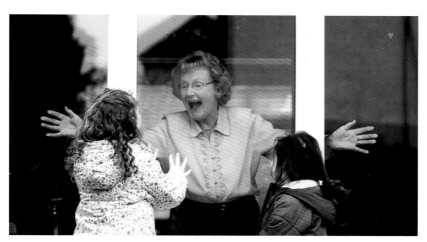

Elena (7) and Lucy (5) Tintori visiting their grandmother Sheela. (*Thomas Honan/ The Irish Times*)

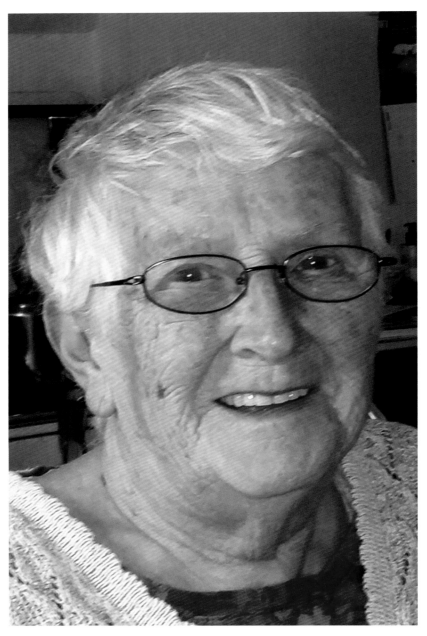

Sheila Murphy, from Clonakilty, West Cork, died following an outbreak at Clonakilty Community Hospital. Her family and all who knew her remember her for her rebellious streak, keen sense of justice and loving nature.

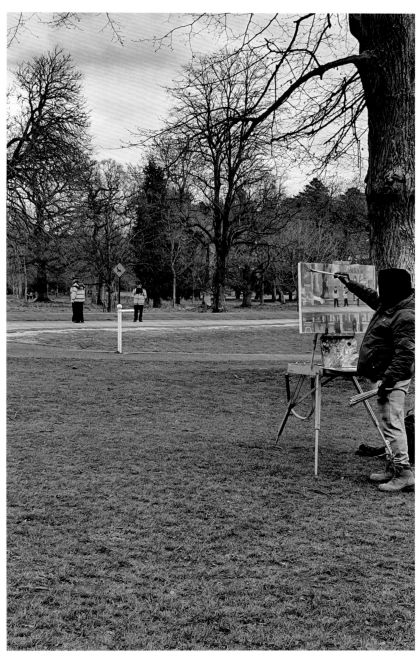

A still life of lockdown: an artist captures a Garda checkpoint in Dublin's Phoenix Park in March 2020.

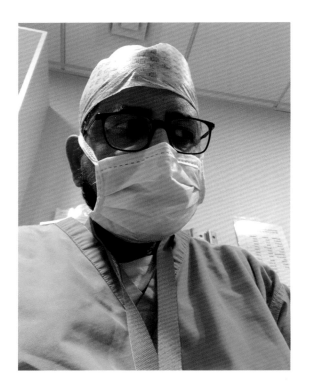

Dr Syed Waqqar Ali, a selfless and brave healthcare worker who was a hero and inspiration to his young family. He died on 21 July 2020.

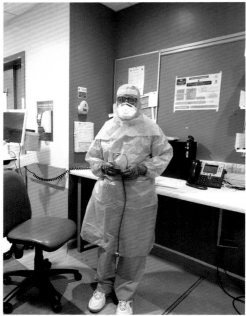

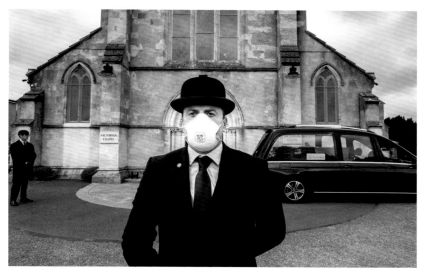

A haunting goodbye. Funeral director Robert Maguire in Mount Jerome, Dublin, where Covid-19 victim John Gallagher was laid to rest. (*Sunday Independent / Mediahuis Ireland - David Conachy*)

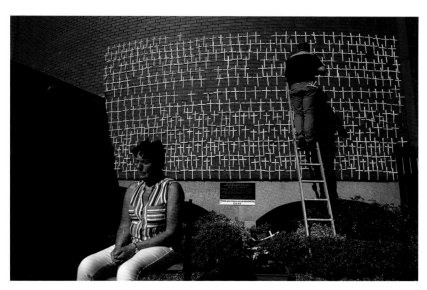

'A wall of crosses and a million tears'. A parishioner prays as crosses are added to Balally Church, Dublin. Each cross represents a life lost to the virus in Ireland. (*Clodagh Kilcoyne/Reuters*)

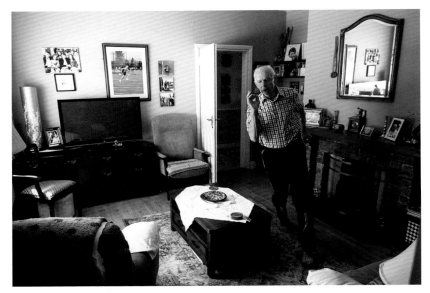

Masters athlete Pat Naughton, 87, trains at home in Nenagh, Co Tipperary. All sporting activity was suspended in the early lockdown, forcing athletes to improvise new training regimens. (*Stephen McCarthy/Sportsfile*)

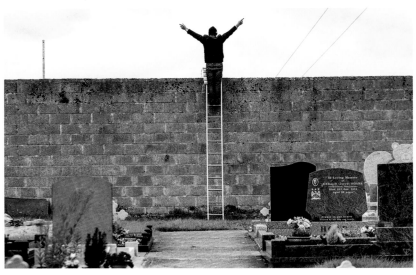

Drastic times meet drastic measures. A fan watches the Roscommon Senior Football Championship Semi-Final from an adjacent graveyard. (*INPHO/James Cromble*)

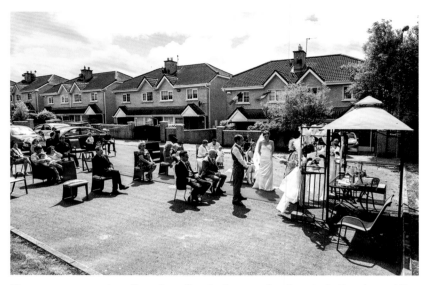

The summer reopening allowed small gatherings to take place, including the wedding ceremony of Tara Leguilloux and Terence Lenihan in Donnybrook, Co Cork. (*Eóin Noonan/Sportsfile*)

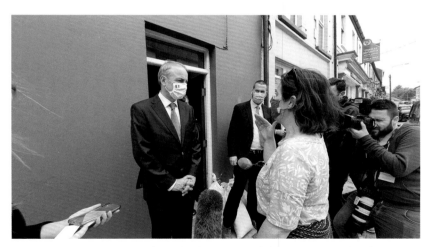

A teacher confronts Taoiseach Micheál Martin in Skibbereen, Co Cork. The nascent coalition was under immediate pressure over confusing guidelines and a series of miscommunications.

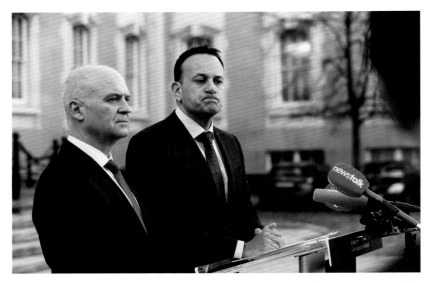

Then-Taoiseach Leo Varadkar and Dr Tony Holohan pause for questions outside Government Buildings. Varadkar's attack on the CMO in October would become a turning point in Ireland's Covid-19 experience. (*PA Images / Alamy Photo*)

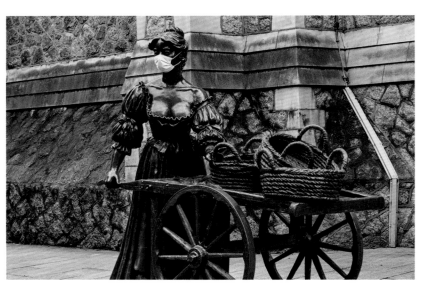

The Molly Malone statue masks up. Ireland, and the western world, was a latecomer to face-coverings. (*Alamy Photo*)

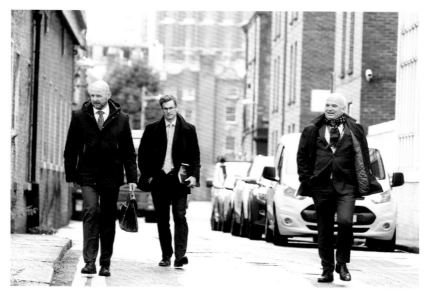

The rift: a returning Tony Holohan leads the NPHET delegation into the Cabinet sub-committee meeting to push for a return to Level 5. The October flashpoint would create a fissure in the relationship between the health officials and the Government they advised. (*Sasko Lazarov/Rollingnews.ie*)

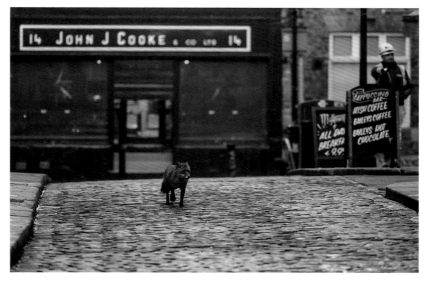

January 2021 brought the worst of the pandemic to Ireland and the renewed lockdown left town and city centres deserted. Dublin's urban foxes became a much more common sight. (*Artur Widak/NurPhoto/PA Images*)

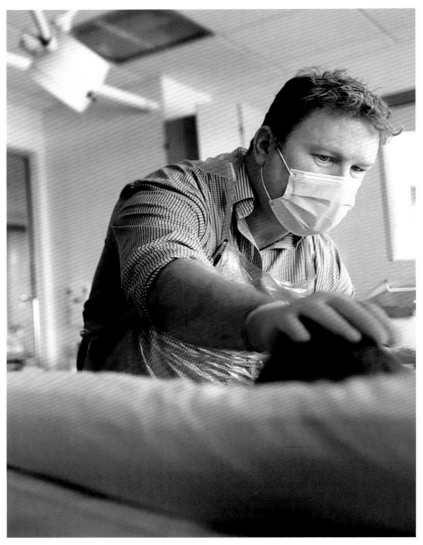

'If we see the same tomorrow, we're done for.' Dr Colman O'Loughlin in the ICU at the Mater Hospital, Dublin. Mortality 'nearly doubled' in intensive care in the third wave. (*Sunday Independent / Mediahuis Ireland - David Conachy*)

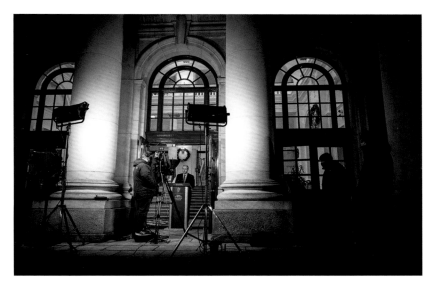

Micheál Martin, from a deserted Government Buildings, announces renewed Covid restrictions on December 30th. His coalition's handling of the Christmas reopening will be debated, and criticised, for years. (*Julien Behal/Rollingnews.ie*)

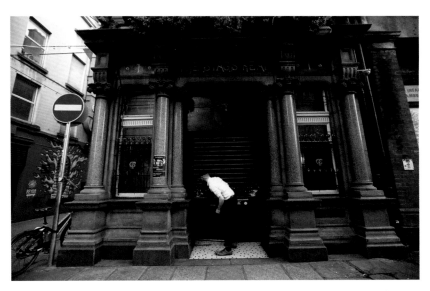

A barman closes the Stag's Head pub in Dublin on Christmas Eve. It would be the start of the longest lockdown in Europe as Ireland's third wave began to bite. (*Sam Boal/ Rollingnews.ie*)

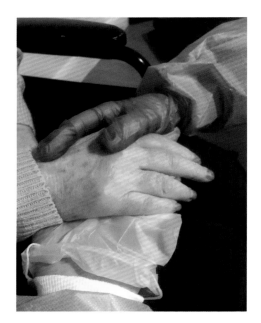

Noreen Butler is visited
by her daughter Judith,
after nine long months of
separation at Christmas 2020.
It was to be the last time they
would hold hands.

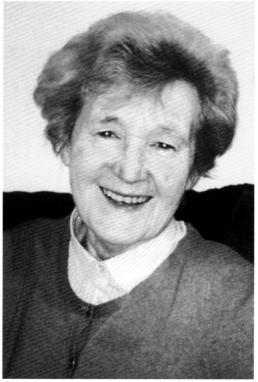

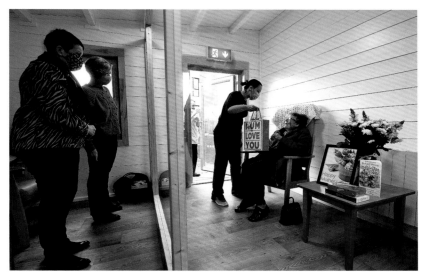

Sisters Carmel Matthews and Rita Ray visit their mother Rosalyn Redmond in an outdoor visiting cabin with perspex divider on Mother's Day 2021. Hugs were still not advised, more than a year in to the pandemic. (*Clodagh Kilcoyne/Reuters*)

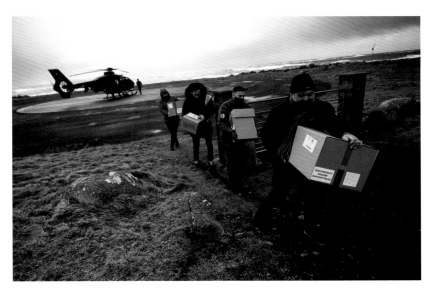

Dr Kevin Quinn, Arranmore Island's GP for more than 30 years, battles the conditions as he and his daughter, clinical nurse Aoife, take delivery of Moderna vaccines by Defence Forces helicopter. (*Clodagh Kilcoyne/Reuters*)

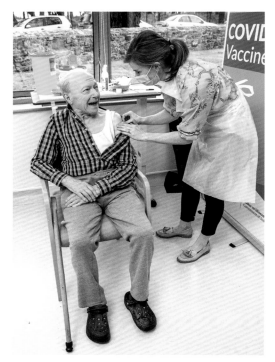

'Hopefully it will help me see my two grandchildren again'. A smiling Michael Farrelly, aged 89 from the South Circular Road gets his first dose at St Mary's Hospital in the Phoenix Park, Dublin, one of the facilities hit hardest by the first wave.

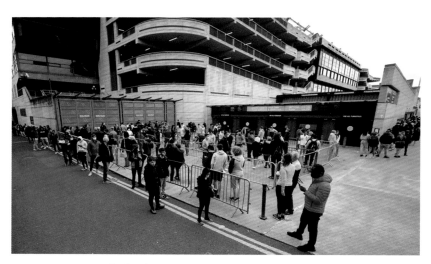

2 August 2021: Hundreds of young people queued for up to two hours outside Croke Park, Dublin on 'walk-in weekend'. 16 and 17 year olds accounted for half of those vaccinated over the Bank Holiday weekend. (*PA Images / Alamy Photo*)

page. The emotions of so many people that had been expressed to her rushed to her head. She stood in her wedding dress, being fitted as she typed furiously, filing copy on her iPhone.

Back in Dublin, she was booked into the hairdressers and filed more copy there. An older woman sitting next to her, getting a blue rinse done, caught her eye.

'Oh my God, did you hear about those politicians in Galway?'

Aoife replied with a smile: 'Yeah, I heard about it.'

She laughed to herself. She knew then that the politics of the pandemic had changed for ever. *Ní neart go cur le chéile*; 'We're all in this together.' Not any more.

* * * *

In Government, mistrust was sown early on. Relying on virtual meetings broke up any chance of building natural chemistry. There was scant opportunity for ministers of different political stripes to mingle over a pint or a coffee. Things quickly turned uneasy.

'You had three parties watching each other,' says one of the Fianna Fáil ministers. 'Bar the Taoiseach himself, the rest of us didn't have any Cabinet experience. The other crowd did. You'd look at Fine Gael's ministers and you'd remember that just weeks ago they were wondering "Jesus, will we call another election because we're so popular."' Tribal instincts were difficult to shake.

'The first couple of months were very difficult,' says one key member of the Fine Gael setup. Any hope of the new coalition pulling itself together to steer us through the pandemic appeared to be fading as case numbers once again crept upwards.

On 18 August, at a hastily organized Cabinet meeting to discuss rising infections, Varadkar's frustrations became clear. He seethed, demanding to know why there was no sub-committee to thrash out the recommendations put forward by Ronan Glynn and NPHET rather than cobbling together a Cabinet meeting to give a knee-jerk response. 'If we keep doing business like this, we won't be doing business for very long,' he declared.

Varadkar and Martin were not easy bedfellows. Animosity between the pair pre-dated the election. They had warred with each other in the Dáil and vowed not to go into Government with each other, Varadkar infamously likening Martin to a 'sinning priest' in 2019, remarks he would be forced to apologize for. In the past Martin had described Varadkar as a 'prickly' man with an 'authoritarian streak' and very sensitive to criticism. They are all charges that many in Fianna Fáil would recognize in their own leader. In many ways, they are similar. Both are fond of clean living and healthy routines; Varadkar was a regular in the gym while Martin would be known to criticise the eating habits of snacking journalists, once tutting that the bunch of grapes being enjoyed by a political correspondent were 'balls of sugar'. Varadkar wasn't used to taking direction from his new colleague. After early engagements in the Sycamore Room, Varadkar would often turn left towards the Taoiseach's office, before sheepishly turning back to the right towards his new office, the Tánaiste's room.

The Tánaiste wasn't just struggling to get used to his new digs. Micheál Martin's long background in 'Fianna Fáil-style' governance saw the Tánaiste dragged into lengthy social dialogues with interest groups, a multitude of sub-committees and all manner of other engagements. The pair, alongside Eamon Ryan, could spend upwards of twenty hours in rooms together every week. Varadkar's reign had focused more on what his aides described as a 'presidential' approach.

The first weeks of union in government were anything but harmonious. The virus was sneaking back into Irish communities too.

On 10 July, the Taoiseach announced that face coverings would, at long last, become compulsory on public transport. Many scientists had been begging for a long, long time for the measure to be introduced. Professor Luke O'Neill of Trinity College Dublin had, since the spring, been pushing studies on growing evidence around wearing masks. Up until the early summer, NPHET and international agencies went so far as to push people away from masks, warning them that incorrect use or considering them a 'magic shield' would be dangerous. Early adopters, walking into supermarkets, would be the targets of stray, quizzical looks from fellow shoppers.

At an earlier meeting between Holohan, Glynn and the Taoiseach, Micheál Martin pushed them on face coverings. Martin's sister, who lives in Singapore, was flat out ringing and texting – 'Why are you guys not doing masks?' Holohan and Glynn told the Taoiseach that it was a different culture in Asia. 'There is a point to that', concedes Martin, but 'the evidence was there'. Singapore, Hong Kong and Taiwan had mask mandates early in the pandemic, their experience shaped by previous infectious disease scares. By March, in some of the most densely populated areas in the world, they had fewer than a thousand Covid cases combined.

For Luke O'Neill, Ireland was among the countries slow to act unless the scientific data was brought to a copper-fastened consensus. 'You need strong leadership to say the evidence is there and strong enough to take action. Ireland waited too long until other people jumped on these things first.'

The slow movement on masks is a regret harboured by many in Government and some of NPHET's membership. It's a matter of regret too among journalists, including me, that we didn't push harder on the subject as the data points grew. The importance of face coverings is a lesson that has been re-learned over multiple pandemics, dating back to the plague. It appears the uptake was all too late once more in the time of

Covid. The near-universal adherence by the public following their introduction showed that the lack of trust that they would be worn properly and safely was unjustified.

Phase Four of the reopening schedule was delayed, first on 15 July and again on 4 August, with 'wet pubs' not serving food remaining shut while the €9 'substantial meal' offerings allowed the remainder to keep trading.

Cabinet grumbled, with Fine Gael's battle-weary contingent the most aggrieved. There were tensions, says Micheál Martin, who struggled to keep Varadkar's increasingly impatient ministers onside. 'They would have said "we've done the reopening, let's keep going with travel and all of that" and we're saying "hang on a second now", you know?'

Things had begun to slide, in spite of their reservations. On 15 August, 200 new cases were confirmed – the most in a single day since the reopening began back in May. Meat factory outbreaks in Kildare, Laois and Offaly brought home the inevitable. For a government that had silently hoped to never again bring in new restrictions, the decision to impose a 'Midlands lockdown' was a 'sickener' for morale.

More national restrictions followed on 18 August. The message was starting to falter as the restrictions became more difficult to follow. Restaurants were curfewed to 11.30 p.m, people were told to go back to working from home, sports were returning behind closed doors and gatherings indoors and outdoors were capped at six and fifteen people respectively. The GAA was among the groups peeved by the restrictions, effectively calling out Ronan Glynn and asking him to perform a presentation for them.

The new Health Minister wasn't winning friends either. A series of unsteady media performances by Stephen Donnelly was topped off in an infamous interview with Zara King of Virgin Media News, in which he compared the risks of sending kids to school during the pandemic to the risks of children bouncing on trampolines. It was viral fodder, the Minister's satisfied smile adding to the cringe factor. It was an unforced error the Government struggled to shake off. The minister, by many accounts, is still not over it, pointing to it as an example of being hard done by in the media. Donnelly still stands over the point in casual conversations, although he concedes that perhaps he should have referred to riding a bicycle rather than jumping on a trampoline.

Days later, as questions continued to mount about the Golfgate controversy, he was landed in a difficult situation as his press adviser Colette Sexton stepped in to try to deflect questions about the matter. Donnelly privately admitted that communications was becoming a weak spot. But the question marks over his tenure would not go away as the trajectory of the virus continued to climb higher and higher.

With fissures cracking the Government apart and Fine Gael increasingly exasperated with NPHET, the coalition and its public health advisers would soon find themselves on a collision course that would come to define their relationship.

Chapter 12: The Blindside

Professor Philip Nolan was pacing around the Royal Hospital in Kilmainham with his phone clamped to his ear. It was the first weekend of October, and NPHET was scrambling with texts and calls flying in all directions. After three months, Dr Tony Holohan was back in the frame. It was clear that a swift change in direction was coming.

'Here's what I think he's going to do …'

'Well, this is where we are …'

'It's likely to require more action.'

Spending the weekend in Schull in West Cork, Dr Colm Henry turned to his wife and said they should head out to a restaurant for dinner. Why? 'Well, we won't be out again for a while.'

Holohan, deferentially known as 'The Boss' by many of his senior colleagues in NPHET, including Deputy CMO Ronan Glynn, was concerned about the virus's re-emergence. He had been for quite some time.

In August, despite everything going on at home, the CMO was keeping a close eye on proceedings. Privately, he felt the focus had become too centred on three counties – Kildare, Laois and Offaly – and not the country as a whole. It's understood that Holohan texted Glynn at the time offering counsel. 'Stick to your principles, stand up to the political pressure, make the calls. Don't be afraid.'

Holohan was scheduled to return to his desk at the Department of Health on Monday, 5 October, but things were moving quickly. Far more quickly than anyone might have imagined. On Thursday, 1 October, Glynn led a NPHET meeting that came to a consensus: Ireland did not need to move up to Level 3 restrictions. We would stay at Level 2. Further action couldn't be ruled out in the future, with the Acting CMO raising strong concerns about the growth in clusters and outbreaks.

On the same day as Glynn's NPHET meeting, news of Holohan's impending return broke, flashing across journalists' screens as an *Irish Times* news alert as they waited to pepper Minister Stephen Donnelly with questions at a briefing.

The minister's first reaction was one of praise and joy, speaking about looking forward to working alongside the CMO, of whom he remarked, 'sure he became a national hero when Covid arrived'.

But there would be no hero's welcome. The weekend that followed would rock the relationships between the CMO, the Minister for Health, the Government and the HSE to their core.

Holohan arrived at the Department of Health ahead of schedule on the Friday, meeting with Ronan Glynn to review the data. By then, the cases from Thursday and Friday were available. 'This just isn't good enough,' he said as they scrolled through the HPSC data. In the previous two weeks, Ireland had had 2,000 confirmed cases. In the week up to Wednesday, 30 September, there were 1,100 cases. By the Sunday, the number was up to 3,000 cases.

'Certainly, Ronan knew and was deeply concerned about the direction things were going,' says Professor Philip Nolan. 'We had been engaging with Government to say they needed to take radical action pretty quickly.' Glynn and Nolan were in constant contact, buzzing each other four times over the course of Saturday, comparing notes on how they would navigate Holohan's return. In Kilmainham, Nolan peeled off from the friends he was out for a walk with to handle the relentless calls. 'Where are we?'; 'This is going to be bad'; 'What should we do?' All the while, Holohan was also contacting his most trusted advisers, war-gaming what needed to be done. This was a whirlwind.

Most members of the group knew that Holohan would immediately push for increased restrictions, but there were 'significant differences of opinion' about the message and how to deliver it to Government.

As one senior NPHET person involved in the ring-arounds put it: 'What was going on in those phone calls was kind of "How are we going to deal with this?" and the strong advice we were trying to get to Tony was to slow down and not make any hasty decisions. "You're going too fast, too hard and you just need to take a breath. You're doing the right thing but you're going about it the wrong way."'

Over the course of Saturday, Holohan decided that there would need to be an emergency meeting of NPHET on Sunday. There were gulps of trepidation at the prospect. In political circles, the rumblings around Tony Holohan's return were met with a sense of panic. 'Tony arrived back like a storm,' says Green Party leader Eamon Ryan. Jokingly, TDs texted each other: 'He's coming back to lock us down.' Little did they know.

The question of how to keep the Government in the loop was key. Some advised Holohan to skip past the Health Minister and ring the alarm directly with Taoiseach Micheál Martin. Holohan, however, was adamant that he would stick to the chain of command. 'That's the fucking Minister's job.' What was the feeling among some of those who told him to bypass Stephen Donnelly and go straight to the Taoiseach? 'Never send a boy on a man's errand.' For Philip Nolan, 'That was one point of the pandemic where communications between Government and NPHET completely broke down.'

Tony Holohan texted the Minister for Health, saying he was concerned about where things were headed. Stephen Donnelly at this point, according to sources close to the Minister, thought holding the Sunday NPHET meeting was prudent. He didn't, however, inquire as to what the outcome of that meeting might mean by way of a lockdown recommendation. This, for many NPHET participants, remains hard to understand. 'Where the Jaysus was the Minister?' asks one NPHET member.

The Taoiseach was all but in the dark, having only just received a text from his minister that afternoon. Micheál Martin, out on an hour's walk around the marina in Cork City, called Donnelly. 'He was getting the sense that it could go to Level 4 or Level 5,' the Taoiseach said.

'Jesus,' Martin sighed into the phone.

Sunday came. Donnelly checked in with Holohan, 'just to see what was going on'. NPHET members believe that, during the conversation between Donnelly and Holohan, Donnelly himself asked to sit in on the NPHET meeting. As his predecessor, Simon Harris, had found out, there was no way Holohan would allow the meeting to go ahead with the minister in it. 'Nothing personal,' he was assured.

At this moment, Holohan told Donnelly that it was likely that further restrictions would be recommended off the back of the meeting – putting the prospect of a Level 4 or 5 recommendation firmly on the table.

The meeting began. It was tense. In West Cork, Dr Colm Henry struggled to connect to the video meeting from a car park and was flitting in and out of signal. Henry was one NPHET member known to harbour reservations about the speed at which the CMO was moving, without prior engagement or groundwork with the Government. Did he express that concern at the time? 'I couldn't actually because I had big connection difficulties on that particular meeting. Ultimately, at the end of it, there is a strong public health entity in NPHET that is very powerful. That's their business and they persuaded the rest of us that it was the right thing to do.'

There was a bit of 'to and fro', but everyone noted their concern at rising incidence among older age groups, hospital admissions and a frightening rise in clusters in nursing homes. 'It wasn't a hard sell,' says one leading member of NPHET, 'it wasn't a sense of Tony going round the place beating people up with a fucking baseball bat.' In the end, the decision of the meeting was Level 5 restrictions, a return to a full national lockdown, for a period of four weeks.

There were suspicions in political circles about the running of NPHET meetings. Word leaked out to political operatives about the 'autocratic' nature of the Chief Medical Officer's tenure. There was certainly a difference between how Holohan ran NPHET meetings and how Ronan Glynn did.

'If you say something stupid, you'll know you've said it with Tony,' says Professor Philip Nolan, 'you probably won't know it with Ronan. They just have different ways of absorbing what everybody is telling them and turning it into a proposal. At the end of the day somebody has to say, "Here's what we're going to do." Tony does it more bluntly and more directly. I think people would think that Ronan is inclusive and takes everybody's views on board, and Tony might have formed a view on the way in. Actually, it's just that they're absorbing the information in different ways.'

Another longstanding member, who had been in the trenches under both men, summed it up: in their view, Ronan is 'absolutely much more collaborative, much more conciliatory. He'd bring everybody together. He did remarkably well taking over in very difficult circumstances and I gather himself and Tony get on well though. He's being groomed for the big job by Tony.'

After the meeting, Holohan and Glynn briefed Minister

Donnelly and the interim Secretary General, Colm O'Reardon. It was a short meeting, before the formal letter putting forward the recommendations was submitted to Government, but this is when the recommendation to bring the country back to a Level 5 lockdown was put to the Minister.

Holohan contacted Liz Canavan in the Department of the Taoiseach to try to organize a briefing with the senior officials in the civil service. It was all too late for that. The matter had already risen above their pay grade.

What was fast becoming a challenging situation was about to be made all the worse. The NPHET recommendation was leaked to the national media. The nine o'clock news, flash notifications and headlines warning of a return to the lock and key of restrictions were everywhere. It filled the nation with a Sunday night dread like never before. Traders worried that they wouldn't be able to open up shop in the morning, families worried that schools would be shut.

'We hit the roof at the NPHET recommendation,' says one senior minister, who was part of the Cabinet sub-committee who would meet to discuss it. 'We hit the roof. It came out of absolutely nowhere. We really felt strongly that NPHET had landed us in it. They had landed the Government in having to make an incredibly hard set of decisions that we just weren't set up to do.'

To the ministers, this was a 'bounce'. The government's senior civil servants and ministers suspected the leak was a ploy by Holohan and NPHET to force the government into immediate action. Sitting at home in his apartment in Castleknock, Varadkar was fielding calls and texts from his party's ministers. 'We were astounded,' he says. The vast majority of Fine Gael's TDs had heard about it first on the news, with many straight on to their leader for clarity.

Eamon Ryan was getting the sense of immediate pushback from the machine of government. 'There was a sensitivity in the political system because we were responding to media rather than a report and analysis.' As the party leaders discussed how to handle the recommendation, Ryan felt a sense of betrayal seething among his colleagues. 'We're being bounced into stuff here using the media,' he said. 'I think that coloured everything as well as the speed of locking everything down.'

Finance Minister Paschal Donohoe, usually one of the most even-tempered in Cabinet, was livid. His colleague at the Department of Public Expenditure and Reform, Michael McGrath, was said to be equally furious. McGrath has a questioning mind. Before joining the new Government, he would often approach reporters with questions that had struck him or his wife while they watched the press conferences. He was keenly aware of the dangers of the virus, but he wasn't minded to throw thousands of people back onto the PUP overnight.

With furious politicians left scrambling, fielding angry texts and calls from constituents late on Sunday evening, TDs and party members raced online to point the finger at the doctors, whom they suspected of becoming more and more political, or 'drunk on power', as one junior minister described it. 'Cabinet was being usurped,' said another Fianna Fáil minister.

The CMO, Deputy CMO and members of NPHET deny leaking. 'It was a total stitch-up,' says one key player. 'It was about trying to turn the discussion from being one about "do we need to do this stuff?" into one about "look at these fuckers there. They've ideas above their station. They're out there leaking; they're playing political games."'

NPHET, whatever about the protests from Holohan and Glynn, does leak. Its discussions have found their way into the national press and news bulletins. It's clear that both Chief Medical Officers are stung by how it's come about. Glynn admits: 'Clearly, we've had leaks from NPHET and that's public record. I don't know who it is or why they're doing it but I think they've done a significant disservice to the public health response.' Holohan took the same view, noting, like Glynn, that the leaks started last summer while he was on leave. 'Five or six times', he says, he's had to remind everyone logging on to a NPHET discussion about the importance of following procedure. According to people attending those meetings, the two CMOs have effectively gone around the table making it crystal clear that leaks are damaging and undermine everyone at the table and everyone who participates in the process. And yet the practice has continued.

Leo Varadkar has been tagged as being a leaker. In the weeks to come, the hashtag #LeoTheLeak would become a regular tending topic over his disclosure of a confidential GP contract to a friend. Varadkar appears to be one of few in government who will even entertain the possibility that the leak could have come from the government side. 'I, to this day, do not know how it appeared on the news. The general view is that it may have leaked from NPHET and NPHET does leak. Other people say it leaked from Government and Government does leak. I don't know where it came from but the vast majority of ministers certainly heard it on the news. I knew it was coming at that point. We were astounded.'

The letter setting out NPHET's recommendations hit the media about twenty minutes after it was sent. One strong defence from the NPHET side is that only two members of the team had access to the letter and they were Holohan and Glynn themselves, neither noted leakers. Social media revved up with shock at the prospect of a return to weeks of lockdown. Word even reached Downing Street.

A lot has been made of a phone call between the Taoiseach and British Prime Minister Boris Johnson that weekend. The call came when the UK Government became aware of the recommendation from NPHET to move things to Level 5. The story goes that Johnson was very concerned about the situation in Ireland – and the divergence in approaches that would result between the Republic and the North. The call itself actually came when the Taoiseach was in the pharmacy. As Micheál Martin took the call, he pressed a finger to his ear to make sure he heard everything Johnson was saying. 'I was in there for a reason. Just buying something, a passport photo or something. He was ringing pro forma on the recommendation.' It ended up being a short exchange of information: what the process would be in Ireland; the level of concerns in both jurisdictions about the second wave; and a mutual agreement that more focus would be needed north of the border.

On Monday, it was time for the meeting itself. NPHET on Merrion Street arrived in a trio – Holohan, Glynn and Nolan – with the projections to justify their stance. Their footsteps echoed through the marble entrance hall. They had been in this foxhole before, but not in these circumstances. On another of these seminal days, on a staircase at Government Buildings, Holohan turned to Nolan, with whom he had interned as a trainee doctor in St Vincent's in Dublin, and said, 'There are many times we'd probably have walked together up a stairs in Vincent's ... did we ever think we'd end up in a situation like this together?' This, of all their moments together over the course of 2020, would be among the most daunting.

As the meeting began, the NPHET members could sense this was not going to be an easy ride. NPHET's concerns were addressed, while the HSE's CEO Paul Reid explained what was happening in hospitals. The NPHET contingent was dismayed when Reid gave his presentation. 'We're coping' was his message. This gave reassurance to the Government that they didn't need to be swept along by Holohan's warnings. To members of NPHET, both within and outside the room, the fact that Reid had, as they saw it, gone to bat for the Government was a body blow and deepened a feeling that he wasn't an ally in the public health arena. To them, the HSE's CEO was focusing on the present, not on a dangerous future that could threaten those same hospitals. A nickname has stuck to Reid among some members of NPHET and the HSE's senior management team – 'the Professor', because of his fondness for regurgitating informed expressions of public health wisdom from his colleagues.

Reid himself says that he was 'shocked and surprised' by the recommendation put forward by NPHET. 'You know, the Sunday, I obviously was alerted the meeting was happening and I was saying "Jesus ..." and then a decision is taken on Sunday night and I'm going "fucking hell".'

On the same day as the Cabinet sub-committee meeting, Reid tweeted, 'There's obvious concerns about the trends on #COVID19. But we also know the impacts of severe & regular restrictions in society on the public health, wellbeing, mental health and the economy. Level 5 recommendation to Government has to be considered in this context too.' The tweet did not go down well with NPHET members, who felt it ignored an obvious trend that even the most rigid of lockdown sceptics in government had to accept was troubling. Senior management figures in the HSE do admit there was a strong resistance to NPHET at the time, shaped by the sense that Holohan was wielding too much power and looked upon the HSE as subordinates under his control, pawns on the board to deploy as he saw fit.

The NPHET members had a sense that the sub-committee was 'going to make a bad decision here'. The bad feeling in government circles even went so far as to take issue with the formatting of the Holohan letter. The emphatic underlining of turns of phrase like 'now' and the ruling out of a graduated response felt, to some in the coalition parties, like a broader part of 'the bounce'.

The sting was most acutely felt in the Taoiseach's chair. Micheál Martin was blindsided by the move. So too was Martin Fraser. As the meeting rolled on, the Taoiseach cut a dejected figure. Senior officials and members of the Government present strongly sensed that he was personally wounded by the recommendation coming out of the blue. He angrily shook his head at questions and answers. He found it jarring that this recommendaton, life-changing as it was for thousands of households across the country, had been allowed to go so far without any direct contact being made with him.

Martin, whatever about the poor state of communications from the Government at times during the pandemic, had been in regular contact with people managing the health response. He'd regularly call Tony Holohan, Ronan Glynn or Paul Reid from the back of his car on the road from Dublin or Cork asking for their take on whatever the latest development might be, or what other countries were adding to their armoury to tackle the virus. The fact that he himself was now sore over the recommendation was a conflict the Government and their advisers could have done without. 'We could see it in the room. He was upset. He hadn't been done the courtesy of being warned this was coming,' says one witness.

The NPHET delegation knew the argument was already lost. A furious Paschal Donohoe let them have it. 'We can't go on like this,' he said, looking down the table at the trio. 'We cannot go on like this.' The Finance Minister told the meeting that Holohan and his crew had completely lost sight of what the Government was asking the public to do. He said the Level 5 recommendation broke the 'Living With Covid' levels scheme, agreed only weeks prior to the meeting, when Holohan was on leave. Donohoe also worried how the European Central Bank would react to the news that Ireland would stand alone in the EU as the only member state once again locked up.

Donohoe, while appreciative of the human cost of Covid, was concerned about the bottom line. Members of both Leo Varadkar's and Micheál Martin's Governments said you could always sense the weight of balancing the books on Donohoe.

'Paschal, not unreasonably, thinks he saved the economy. He has strong ties in Europe, he always said that things would be okay because of his relationship with Eurogroup.' It's a claim also levelled by Shane Ross, when he was in Cabinet. 'I remember one day him saying to me when I was going in for more money for tourism and him saying, "Look, this is all terrible but we'll come out of it. Why? Because of me. People in Europe trust me."'

The meeting rolled on and on with participants squinting at slides, and folding arms in crumpled shirts. The sparks that flew threatened to combust entirely. Holohan was told, in a revealing aside, that the Government would be unfairly blamed for any rise in new deaths if it decided against going to full Level 5 and that NPHET had dumped the coalition in this 'unviable' position. Philip Nolan's modelling of what could lie around the corner was openly disparaged. At one point, Martin Fraser gave Nolan an unabashed 'bollocking' in front of the meeting, later apologising to him over the phone. Ministers, both in the room and outside it, contemplated whether or not NPHET should have been wound up in the summer. Some were more frustrated with the growing perception of 'politicians versus doctors' and how the showdown would look to a worried public.

The NPHET members were dismissed. The Cabinet sub-committee breathed a sigh of relief and put their heads together, wondering what to do next.

For Paschal Donohoe, one of the biggest factors in not going with NPHET's advice – the first time the Government instigated a serious breakaway from the recommendations of its public health advisers – was the fact that the Budget was round the corner. He wanted a message of 'certainty and confidence' for the public. And this, to his mind, was anything but. Many in the political sphere had an underlying resentment towards Holohan. It was growing. Some admit there was an element of jealousy about the CMO's national icon status the previous

185

spring. He had become a fixture in households, a paternalistic figure offering reassurance when the virus was frightening and new. His approval numbers far outstripped any politician's. This, to borrow a phrase from politics across the water, was a move to 'Take Back Control'.

Senior ministers present had a good read of the room. One new minister said that Martin Fraser and Robert Watt in particular weren't for budging. 'They weren't shy about shutting things down, I think, but I think they felt they were being bumped into it, bounced into it and they were sensitive to the economic interests. Robert Watt was raging – "What are you doing?"'

As the Taoiseach of a government that had already seen its share of controversies and calamities, Micheál Martin had hit a new level of frustration. Sitting in his office in Government Buildings, he clasps his hands together, thinking deeply about the impact that tempestuous weekend had. 'NPHET already seemed to have made up its mind without any preparatory work. You have to prepare the ground in all things.'

Martin personally spoke to Tony Holohan, with disappointment written across his face. 'I would have appreciated a call.' In a separate moment of the interview, the Taoiseach gave an indication as to why he might have been so upset at being bypassed. He explained why he calls the CMO or the HSE chief on occasion himself. 'It's probably part of my make-up but also, something gets lost in the messaging sometimes when it's third-party or second-party or hearsay,' he says. 'The first line of communication, you're hearing it from the source. It's the thing of the historian having to get to the primary source of something, you know?'

Whether or not that's intended as a subtle slight against the Health Minister, it's clear that direct engagement with the Taoiseach would have swept away the notion of the Government being 'blindsided'. Holohan, it's understood, felt bad about personally offending the Taoiseach but in subsequent conversations with NPHET colleagues has told them it would have led to more trouble at the time. 'If Martin Fraser found out I was ringing the Taoiseach just off my own bat ... they already think we have ideas above our station,' is how Holohan expressed his view to his inner circle. It was a tactical misstep by the veteran public health doctor. He didn't do something that would have been outside the boundaries of protocol but would have been very wise. It's a mistake that blemished his standing in the corridors of power.

As one NPHET member put it: 'He would have been entirely within his rights just to cut across everyone and call the Secretary to Government and the Taoiseach to say: "I'm back, I've formed the view that we're not moving quickly enough and I'm going to advise you in forty-eight hours' time that we need to move more quickly."'

'I have to honestly say I think October was one of those points where Tony's strong style got the better of him,' admits Philip Nolan. 'It was right. Urgent action was necessary but I do think the whole process of how advice was delivered to government could have been better handled.'

Professor Nolan, one of Holohan's closest colleagues on the NPHET team, is frank about the disaster that weekend turned out to be. 'It wasn't from NPHET but from somewhere around the system, the news of advice around another lockdown was leaked. That was really quite damaging. The sense from me anyway, that despite the urgency we might be moving too quickly in terms of how our advice was formed and delivered. I guess that was my fundamental view. Rather than meet and deliver advice to Government, which would surprise them, the correct step was to engage with Government, express the concern that the situation is deteriorating very rapidly and they might need to prepare themselves for additional measures. It just played into the hands of people who didn't want to hear the bad news.'

Some members of the sub-committee are philosophical about the flare-up, satisfied with the clipping of NPHET's wings, claiming it was something that simply needed to happen. 'NPHET as an institution were still new,' says one prominent minister, 'perhaps not at all accustomed to the public eye ... but you can't do that to a Government. We are elected, we live and die by the people's votes, we have the responsibilities of governing. And you cannot bounce a Government.'

The Taoiseach made a short statement to the media after the full Cabinet came together to reject the recommendation. Level 3 was as far as the Government was prepared to go. Ministers at the meeting bristled about the situation. Again, a number of ministers across the parties say that Micheál Martin and Martin Fraser were the most visibly put out. Minister for Foreign Affairs Simon Coveney says: 'NPHET don't actually have to, but we have to factor in, you know, the increase in PUP payments, supports for businesses if we're about to shut them down. You know, there's a whole load of knock-on consequences in terms of cost and planning and reassurance and support that the Government has to plan for.'

Rather than calming the situation and moving on collectively, the Tánaiste was about to drive the newfound mistrust to a new depth. That Monday night, Tánaiste Leo Varadkar arrived in RTÉ for an appearance on *Claire Byrne Live*. He was frustrated, tired and ready to let his feelings be known. He was led into the RTÉ studios by Jon Williams, the Managing Director of RTÉ News and Current Affairs. What followed was one of the Irish pandemic's great turning points.

Varadkar told the nation that the NPHET recommendation 'came out of the blue'. It 'hadn't been thought through and there hadn't been prior consultation.' Across the country, Twitter timelines lit up at what was unfolding. The Tánaiste outlined all the failings as he perceived them and then he went somewhere else entirely. Varadkar, his anger barely concealed, said that no member of NPHET would ever face 'being on the pandemic unemployment payment', and 'none of them would have to tell somebody that they were losing their job.'

At their homes, NPHET members were watching. Government members were whooping and hollering in raucous delight at the takedown, their WhatsApp groups flooded. One minister admitted he balled his fist watching it: 'Fair play, Leo. Go on, give it socks!' As a journalist, I was watching what was happening from the sofa, bouncing from Twitter to texts to WhatsApp and back again. A text landed, unexpectedly, from a NPHET stalwart who said they were shocked by what Varadkar had said, particularly as a doctor. Though, they added, 'I don't think he set the world on fire in scrubs either.' The emoji of a monkey covering its mouth was attached to the end of the text.

A Rubicon had been crossed. Never before, in the pandemic or otherwise, had a high-ranking member of the Government launched such an aggressive broadside on civil servants. Cillian De Gascun says it 'stung', making him question 'why would you bother doing this? Why would people put themselves forward to do this work and to go out and defend policy and to inform people if you're not getting support from the Government?' He, like others, including people in NPHET and in Government, felt it went beyond what was acceptable and led to a spate of personal attacks on the medics from the public. 'It made things very unpleasant then because all of a sudden, everybody was second guessing everything. It was tough to take,' he says.

One senior NPHET member turned to their partner and said: 'That man knows nothing about me, about my family or my extended family or my friends.' Many civil servants, even outside the Department of Health, were shocked by the attack. Many wondered whether the comment would turn people off careers in the service of the country if a target could be drawn on their backs by one of our most senior politicians in a prime-time interview.

Dr Mary Favier, who was added to NPHET in late March 2020, agrees. She believes that the interview outburst 'fuelled a disgruntlement with restrictions and a sense that NPHET was overreacting and we were all just anxious sort of hissy-fit people.' NPHET was cautious, she believes, 'but look where the lack of caution got us a few weeks later.' One of her colleagues has the same assessment. 'I even thought naively that Tony was in trouble and might need to go. He didn't give a shit.'

Mary Favier has strong views on the row and the uneasy balance of power between Government and NPHET that became so exposed. 'There was an element that was true: this accusation that NPHET was running the country. I think that was by default because of a power vacuum. In the beginning when they were an interim Government it suited them to hide behind NPHET. But once they were in government in June, they allowed NPHET to basically be the only messaging. If they had any sense, they should have absolutely controlled the messaging. They should not have allowed Tony Holohan and others, including myself, have at one stage a daily briefing as if they were the Prime Minister. They should never have allowed briefings that were at prime time for news and repeated.'

It's understood that Tony Holohan watched the programme at home with his family. Confidantes say he personally was well able for the attack, shrugging it off and comparing it to colleagues as a 'clip of a hurl in the middle of a match', but his family, his wife in particular, was upset.

Taoiseach Micheál Martin was still in Government Buildings when the interview was broadcast. He stayed late at work throughout the pandemic, often finishing up after 11 p.m., fully consumed by all aspects of Covid and diligently turning through paper after paper on a to-do pile that never seemed to shrink. The telly was on, according to aides, and he was pacing through the place on the way to the kitchen to make a cup of tea to sustain him. He overheard his Tánaiste's voice. According to people close to Martin, he was very taken aback by what he heard. 'Jesus.'

I ask Martin about this. He says he was 'surprised' by the outburst but that it expressed a frustration that had been brewing in government circles and among parts of the public for quite some time. 'Ultimately, I think too much tension between NPHET and the Government isn't a good thing in the middle of a pandemic.' If the Taoiseach had recognized that tension between Government and NPHET on this scale being played out in public was a bad thing, his recognition certainly didn't stop it.

Most ministers celebrated a win over the medics. But not everyone was happy. Some ministers, including Simon Coveney and Simon Harris, who was still pining over his old Department, privately recoiled at the airing of grievances and the dismissal of a public servant. More than one minister has said they were 'disgusted' with the outburst. According to these ministers, Holohan had returned to do one thing – 'to help us out'. There was a point to what the Tánaiste was saying, but the 'flash of anger' was beyond the pale. 'The very least he deserved in that moment was respect,' one minister says, 'even if we're going to disagree with him as was perfectly within our rights to do.'

It was clear that the situation needed to be brought down to a simmer. Varadkar called Holohan. Back in the first wave, they talked on the phone regularly. The then-Taoiseach would text Holohan on a Saturday or a Sunday asking if he was free to take a call, then call him some unspecified time later, running through his thoughts for an hour or more. They had worked closely together too at the Department of Health when Varadkar held the office of Minister. They had a long relationship and it

191

had been reduced to a public spat in the middle of a national emergency. 'It was a good conversation,' says Varadkar, who, as he told the press the next day, hadn't apologized.

Months later, the Tánaiste is annoyed by how the episode played out publicly. He immediately aims blame at Sinn Féin and the non-Government benches. 'The opposition didn't know whether to agree with us or whether to agree with NPHET. What they did,' he says, 'is quite clever and it's what oppositions often do, is they twist it into my personal attack on "Saint Tony". That actually never happened. I was critical of the decision. I was critical of the advice, how it came about. I didn't make any personal remark about anyone or I didn't mean to.'

On the question of the advice itself, the idea that the Government could have had no clue about the possibility of a quick change in recommendations over the course of that weekend does have some weakness.

In interviews with Virgin Media News and RTÉ's *Six One* on the night of 1 October, Ronan Glynn outlined his concerns about the national picture deteriorating significantly. On being questioned, he told Virgin Media that while the next NPHET meeting was scheduled for early the following week, there was nothing to say that the public health team wouldn't meet again 'in the coming days' to make further recommendations if needs be. 'The recommendations we're making today [to extend Level 2] does not mean we won't be back in the coming days or this day next week to make further and stronger recommendations.'

With Ireland moving up just one notch to Level 3, Holohan's push had failed. Phone calls made to the Chief Medical Officer were blunt. Multiple NPHET members who supported the move to Level 5 felt the handling of the weekend's events were the wrong way to do vital business in the interest of saving lives. The image of Holohan, depicted by one mural in Dublin city centre as Superman, was dented, his invincibility wavering. One phone call in particular was incendiary. HSE Chief Clinical Officer (CCO) Colm Henry phoned Holohan, a man he has known for over thirty years. The respect between the two is steadfast. It's understood that Henry told the CMO he'd blown it. He told the NPHET Chair that he'd always have his back and that he'd stood alongside him on many dark days but there was no escaping the fact he'd made a dog's dinner of the recommendation and how he landed it on Government. Tempers flared. Holohan was furious, telling Henry that he didn't recall hearing any suggestions to do otherwise in the NPHET meeting or at any other point.

Holohan is not one for hindsight criticism or action replays and he is known to have been insulted by the call. Relations between Holohan and Henry were grazed and didn't fully recover in the months to follow.

None of this was good news. What happened in October exposed fully the depth of the rift between the Government and NPHET and between NPHET and the HSE. The events of that weekend, according to multiple high-level sources, would have a major impact on the build-up to Christmas and its fallout.

Ronan Glynn says he understands the perception of Holohan's big return but he believes that even if he had stayed on leave an extra week or two, NPHET would not have got much further through the week without making very significant recommendations. Given the conversations between Glynn, Nolan and other NPHET members before Sunday's meeting and the showdown at Government Buildings, I asked him whether NPHET took the right course of action – whether it was handled the right way. His answer is curt. 'I believe the advice was the correct advice.'

Within two weeks of the rejection of the Level 5 advice and with the second wave unmistakably driving high volumes of infection, NPHET returned, proposing a full lockdown yet again. This time, they had supportive ears from the man who had pilloried them just days before. As one Cabinet sub-committee member put it: 'Leo is interesting. He's very compelling, very capable, highly intelligent … it can change two weeks later in terms of – he's full tilt one way and then full tilt the other way.' His broadside against NPHET 'didn't look very smart now,' the minister says, 'because the numbers went the other way and we had to do it.'

Despite the Government eventually following the NPHET advice on Level 5 two weeks after the initial recommendation, it's clear the two parties still do not see eye to eye on the bruising weekend. Leo Varadkar believes going into lockdown later than Ireland did on 18 October might have prevented what was to follow over Christmas. Tony Holohan is known to believe that going earlier would have driven cases down to a safer level in early December. Micheál Martin thinks we ended up opening up too soon in December. They can't all be right.

This was a weekend where everything changed between NPHET and Government. The united front and shared platform of common purpose was splintered. The frontlines of both groups turned on each other, rather than on the virus. The finger-pointing of blame for leaking and bouncing continues and has flared up since, but never quite so starkly.

'I want to be absolutely clear,' says Philip Nolan, 'I don't want to blame anybody for the events of October. They were a collision between a huge sense of urgency on the CMO's part and a kind of sense of not really wanting to hear the bad news, I think, on behalf of the political system. It's true to say that we, NPHET, as a team try to at least learn from any mistakes we may have made.'

It took time, a long time, for the officials and ministers to rebuild even small elements of the relationship. It wasn't back to normal at all in 2020, even as the Government came to its most crucial decision of the pandemic to date: Christmas.

It would go on to have severe repercussions for the weeks

ahead. Tony Holohan is of the firm belief that not taking action in October had a major impact on January. 'We had an opportunity to intervene with the full set of Level 5 restrictions which we believe, like, should be tried for a four-week period of time,' he says. 'Two weeks later we were back to the same decision point. Things got worse. We needed it then for six weeks instead of four. We needed two more weeks for it, and we started two weeks later so that's a whole four weeks later than we would have been.' Holohan's argument is that Ireland could have regained control over transmission. 'We never really got back to a point of sufficient control.'

When the question was put to the Taoiseach about whether the blazing row affected how his Government viewed NPHET's Christmas recommendations later, he accepts it. 'It may have had. It may have had,' he nods.

Professor Nolan perhaps sums it up most clearly. 'Those tensions, the anger and the suspicion were all still hanging in the air' by the Christmas decision. 'If we hadn't had this row in October, perhaps we might have been listened to.'

Chapter 13: Tired of War

Taoiseach's Office, Government Buildings,
Dublin, 8 November 2020

Micheál Martin was alone on the day of the Munster semi-final. A regular attendee at all Cork matches, not least since his son Micheál Aodh became part of the panel, the Taoiseach had swapped the stands at Páirc Uí Chaoimh for the oak-panelled walls of his office. An office that was occupied for many weekends and long nights. Cork had beaten Kerry in a Hollywood finish, with a last-minute goal by Mark Keane putting Kerry out of the Championship.

Micheál's dad used to bring him along to all the Championship ties with Kerry down through the years, and now his own son was togging out for a famous win. He kicked back at his desk with a bottle of beer, phoning the fellas he'd usually go to the matches with – already making legends out of the men who had lined out for Cork that evening. 'It was a great day,' he remembers fondly, sitting by the same Bossi fireplace he sat beside on that evening of escapism from what had been a suffocating start to his time in government.

Already under pressure from his backbenchers, the decision to take Ireland to a six-week lockdown had only sharpened the daggers. Even ministers who had proudly followed him into Government felt it had been a 'capitulation' to NPHET.

196

'Micheál lost his nerve,' one texted me the day Ireland returned to lockdown with a view to securing a clear run at Christmas.

Being Taoiseach is lonely at the best of times. In the worst of times, it's solitary confinement. Conscious of the risks of multiple members of government being taken out of action by the virus, night after night Micheál Martin ate alone at his desk, the portraits of Collins and de Valera staring down upon him. Martin's weekend ritual was boiling a few eggs and packing a salad with chickpeas, sun-dried tomatoes and sheep's cheese in Cork before jumping in the car back to Dublin, keeping them in the fridge until they were eaten or went off. As he toiled away in the office, his critics circled outside.

'Micheál is a very cautious politician,' says one senior Fianna Fáil TD. 'The political system abandoned control really over to the medics at that stage.' The detractors were emboldened as reams and reams of newspapers were filled with 'Government vs NPHET' headlines and columns. Political commentators called on the Taoiseach, once and for all, to put Tony Holohan and his colleagues back in their box. 'Serious political commentators,' says one senior HSE figure, 'people of huge influence, when they start saying "will you grow a pair of balls", it has a very profound effect on politicians. Of that I have no doubt.'

As the big decisions of October played out in the public eye, more and more questions were being asked about the make-up of the power brokers. No members of the Cabinet sub-committee were women. None of the NPHET delegation of Holohan, Glynn and Nolan was a woman. The HSE CEO, also present for those talks, is a man. Ellen Coyne, columnist and news correspondent with the *Irish Independent*, reflected on the imbalance in October. 'The identikit parade of suits up and down Merrion Street this weekend shows that we must – unfortunately – keep pleading,' she said. Influential women were present for the discussions and the decisions – Micheál

Martin's Chief of Staff Deirdre Gillane, Liz Canavan from the Department, and Eamon Ryan's Joint Chief of Staff Anna Conlan. 'But the main protagonists were all men.'

Coyne noted that the Central Statistics Office had found that lockdown and working from home had a more detrimental impact on women than on men. Eighty per cent of our healthcare workforce are women, and the figure is higher still among public health specialists, but in this health emergency, women's voices in the corridors of power or at lecterns facing the nation were few and far between.

In November, Safe Ireland published its first report into the impact of lockdown on domestic abuse. Between March and August of 2020, 3,450 women contacted domestic violence supports for the very first time. The lack of female representation in the inner circle was also pointed to in a string of oversights from Government: Micheál Martin said it would 'not be fair' on smaller shops, forced to close under Level 5, if supermarkets were permitted to sell 'non-essential' items like baby clothes. On 29 October, Junior Minister Damien English, under questioning from *Prime Time*'s Miriam O'Callaghan, blunderingly described socks and clothes as 'not essential'. Parents across the country were incensed. I asked the Taoiseach about it at a press briefing in the sunshine outside Dublin City Council offices on Wood Quay. Micheál Martin, frustrated at the questions, told me 'you know' people can get clothes if they need them through click-and-collect and delivery, pulling me aside after the press conference to emphasize the point.

It wouldn't be the last time the issue arose. Months later, consultant paediatrician Dr Niamh Lynch would highlight the fact that parents of young and growing kids couldn't size children's shoes for months of the pandemic. No government guidance was available until the end of March 2021.

While the men around politics were discussing telling officials to 'fuck off' or ministers to 'show some balls', women and their partners across Ireland were suffering an enormous burden and hidden grief.

The suffering and isolation of women during lockdown had many painful outcomes, perhaps none more hurtful or traumatic than the restrictions on maternity services.

* * * *

Thirty-one-year-old Louise Byrne and her husband Neil were lost in a bubble of excitement. They had been given the most wonderful surprise of a lifetime on 22 September when Louise found out she was pregnant. 'Oh my gosh,' the couple thought, letting it sink in for a few days before telling Louise's sister and Neil's parents. They were so excited.

The young couple went to the Coombe Women and Infants University Hospital. They had both been born there and wanted to continue the generational family connection.

Six weeks into her pregnancy, on a Friday evening, Louise started bleeding. It was terrifying. She called her sister, who was also pregnant and had a two-year-old child. She gave Louise the emergency number for the Coombe. Louise called it and called it and called it, dialling six times over the course of an hour before getting through. 'Look, I'm very early,' Louise told the midwife on the end of the line, 'I don't know what's going on.'

The helpline, she says, told her not to worry about coming in unless the bleeding worsened. The bleeding continued over the weekend. The helpline again told her that unless she was filling a pad, there was nothing to seriously worry about.

By Sunday morning, disturbed by what had been happening, Louise and Neil took it upon themselves to go directly to the hospital. Louise threw on her Converse trainers and her hoodie. Neil helped Louise through the rain to their 2005 Golf, and they set off for the Coombe. They were lucky to get a parking spot. They arrived inside the front door at a welcome desk.

Like all hospitals, and most offices, the Covid forms were the first duty. The woman at the desk looked at Neil and said, 'He can't come in.' Neil turned and went back to the car park as Louise was sent down to Admissions and then to the Emergency Department.

The first thing she noticed was how empty it was. She sat alone. Shifting on the uncomfortable metal chair, she thought, 'I shouldn't be that long if there's nobody else here.' An hour passed. And then another. And then another. Louise texted Neil, sitting outside in the Golf in a car park full of cars, full of partners not allowed to be with their loved ones. Dozens of cars were outside the Coombe on that miserable morning. The rain bounced off the foggy windscreens as partners waited, with the heaters on, for news from inside.

Louise spent five hours alone, texting Neil. 'All I could think was "What's wrong?" And "I need Neil here with me."' She sat by a wall with her phone charging, playing Candy Crush to distract herself and keeping in contact with Neil. 'I'm really scared,' she texted him. Eventually, she was seen by a doctor.

'When was the last time you had a smear test?'

'I'm not sure. It was a couple of years ago.'

The doctor tried the ultrasound. 'We'll need to do an internal exam.'

Louise was traumatized by the experience. 'I know I'm passing clots; I know I'm losing my baby.'

She was told that her hCG was low, a significant indicator of miscarriage. The doctor told Louise to come back the next day for a blood test and an internal ultrasound in the Early Pregnancy Unit (EPU). Leaving the room, Louise says, 'the doctor said "One in four pregnancies end in miscarriage." That was the last thing she said to me as she was walking out.'

Louise sat with Neil in the car, crying. 'All the dads were still sitting in their cars. People waiting for appointments. We took a few minutes and came home. The next day we went back.'

On the Monday, Neil stayed in the driver's seat and Louise set off for the EPU. She was frustrated when the medic in charge of the internal exam asked her, 'Do you mind if my colleague here watches?' It didn't fully hit her at the time but in the long days that followed, the idea that someone training would be allowed in to observe while she was there without her partner, her rock of support, felt cruel.

The doctors told her to come back in two days for the miscarriage to be confirmed. Louise trudged back to the car. 'You have to pass all these lovely ladies with their lovely bumps sitting there and you know that you're miscarrying. It's ... just to even have someone holding your hand while you're doing that.'

Tuesday was Neil's birthday. It was subdued. Louise and Neil lay in bed for the day watching television and minding their dogs. On Wednesday the call came through to confirm the news they already knew was coming. 'I am now confirming a miscarriage to you.'

Louise knows grief. She had lost her mother nine years before. She wanted to speak about her pain, feeling that 'Irish people in general just don't acknowledge grief.' She wrote to the Lord Mayor of Dublin, to the Health Minister and to the Tánaiste about what she had been through. She posted about it online. She had the support of her sister and Neil; she didn't feel that she had the support of the Government. 'It's just not to the forefront of people's priorities. Particularly in Government. I think a lot of that is to do with the pressure of the public,' she says. 'You've got vintners trying to get pubs open, you've got hairdressers opening and starting GoFundMes. It's just the fact that I can most likely go to a hair salon but if I was to miscarry, I still wouldn't have my husband in the room. It makes me so, so angry.'

Louise and hundreds of others who have felt the impact of the restrictions have taken grave exception to the descriptor 'visiting restrictions' around maternity care. 'They are not visitors. They shouldn't be called visiting hours. It's the partner's child.' Later in the pandemic, protests were held outside many of the country's maternity hospitals, including the Coombe, calling for the restrictions to be loosened as vaccines provided greater cover for staff and patients alike. The Coombe itself was the site of one such protest. All the way through summer, the push continued with many units still not complying with directives from the HSE to ease deeply damaging restrictions.

The burden of Covid on expecting couples as well as families with small children was immense. Dr Niamh Lynch saw children with an array of health issues normally only seen in ageing adults. Chilblains and Raynaud's were diagnosed, resulting from kids being taught in classrooms with open windows, the only means of ventilating crowded classrooms, even on the coldest days. 'I have seen children starve themselves, cut themselves, hit themselves,' she told Twitter. 'I have seen children with tics so severe that they cannot eat or sleep. I have seen toddlers scream in terror at the sight of strangers. I have seen children go from chatterboxes to utterly mute.' Concern about long-term impacts dogged medics at work, and kept worried parents tossing and turning late at night.

* * * *

As Ireland moved through a dreary November, the thoughts of exiting lockdown and enjoying a good Christmas were to the forefront of people's minds. Lockdown was hard and the public were drained. Case counts were not improving as much as health officials had hoped.

'We had to tell them the truth,' says Dr Colm Henry of the HSE, 'our messaging was simply about: "We're all in it together and we can all beat it together." That worked in the summer.

The winter was different. You couldn't lean into that message any more. The population was tired of war.'

Henry, normally based in Cork, holed up in the deserted Hibernian Club on St Stephen's Green in Dublin whenever NPHET and HSE duties required his presence in the capital. His walks back from the Department of Health on Baggot Street were intercepted by urban foxes who had become common sights across the capital as they sought out food on the empty footpaths. The streets, to Colm Henry's mind, didn't feel safe any more. 'The only people you'd see were people you didn't want to meet,' he says. 'I became aware of the security that other people on the street give to you just by their very presence. That did strike me. There was nobody there.'

The Government's decision would come on 26 November and it was fast approaching. The lobbying continued from business groups representing traders who had suffered by far the worst year of their careers, with tens of thousands of long-term staff unemployed.

Politically, the push got louder and louder still. Members of the Dáil, including the Rural Independents' Mattie McGrath, who to much outrage had described the wet pub ban as 'apartheid', advocated for the reopening of bars. Opposition politicians were uneasy at how the Government, now months in office, had seemed to abandon most of the briefings with the Chief Medical Officer and Health Minister which had been a key component of the first wave. Political figures like Sinn Féin's Mary Lou McDonald, Labour's Alan Kelly, the Social Democrats' Róisín Shortall, People Before Profit's Richard Boyd Barrett and more besides were growing ever more frustrated by this. They felt that no effort was being made to properly inform elected representatives of the public health factors behind each of the decisions that governed Irish lives in the second half of 2020.

The finger of blame was pointed at the Taoiseach. 'Micheál

Martin is not good at working with others,' says one opposition leader. 'I find that he has no professional courtesy. I think it's absolutely desperate stuff. It's not conducive to getting a kind of "all of Oireachtas approach" and fostering confidence.' That was not an isolated feeling across the spectrum of Leinster House.

Mary Lou McDonald is one politician who feels that an opportunity to build consensus was missed. While Sinn Féin and Fine Gael have competed for the top spot in the polls throughout the latter half of 2020 and the first half of 2021, she is known to have a workable professional relationship with Leo Varadkar and points to Ireland's unified approach to Brexit as an example of what can happen when the political system is kept informed and encouraged to participate. 'My job is to ensure that whatever course of action we're taking, that I can credibly assure the public that I've done my homework and that we're satisfied that this is the right way forward. It didn't happen and the consequences of that have been profound,' she says.

Chapter 14: A Meaningful Christmas

Department of Health, Miesian Plaza, 26 November 2020

The video link from Government Buildings shut down. The faces of the Taoiseach, the Tánaiste and all manner of ministers, officials and advisers faded from the screen. Zoom calls were almost customary in homes and businesses across Ireland by late November, but none carried the weight of this one.

Tony Holohan, Ronan Glynn and Philip Nolan sat in the boardroom at the Department of Health in silence for a moment, creaking chairs the only sound. After a second's pause, they were all in agreement. Their warning hadn't landed with the Government. They had failed. Privately, they conceded that the political discussion continuing without them at the Cabinet sub-committee less than half a kilometre away would significantly diverge from the path they'd recommended. 'We knew we would be in trouble,' says Glynn. 'It was a question of how much trouble.'

The NPHET members puffed out their cheeks. Holohan had argued that pubs and restaurants should open only for takeaway and delivery over Christmas, fearing super-spreading events when younger people returned to their family homes for Christmas gatherings with older relatives. In their letter to the Health Minister, in their discussions with senior officials and then in the Cabinet sub-committee itself, NPHET argued

205

that if socializing and household mixing took place 'a third wave of disease will ensue much more quickly and with greater mortality than the second'.

Within an hour and a half of their dismissal from the meeting, the members of NPHET beeped their swipe cards through the turnstiles at the ground floor of the Department of Health. Their phones pinged with news alerts. The leaks from the sub-committee had started. The Government was going to go another way. Hospitality, excluding the wet pubs, would be open for 'three busy weekends' in the run-up to Christmas. 'I was very worried about it,' says Holohan. 'We couldn't have created better conditions for what happened over that Christmas and January.'

Philip Nolan was devastated. He had two overwhelming emotions: 'Disappointment and guilt.' In his view, this was a crucial moment the health officials had to get right – they had to stress to the Government how much was at stake, that many, many lives were on the line, that the hospital network had to be protected. They, the advisers, had failed to do it. 'We had failed to persuade government of the gravity of the situation and the need to be much more conservative,' he says. 'It's a real sense of failure. My sense was the blame lay with us rather than with them.' Nolan carried the guilt all through Christmas and for months to follow. It lingers with him still, a knot deep in the stomach. A 'what if?' scenario to end all 'what if?' scenarios. Is there anything else that could have been said or could have been explained that might have changed things?

As the members of NPHET's top table headed home on 26 November, and as the members of the Cabinet sub-committee finished their deliberations, it was the October row that crossed many of their minds. 'If we hadn't had this row back in October, perhaps we might have been listened to …' wondered Philip Nolan as the flurry of tweets from journalists made it clear that the Government had its own plan for Christmas.

The meeting itself had been respectful, polite and far less bruising than the October flashpoint. The old political saying about the 'meeting before the meeting' being the most important one may have been true in the case of the Christmas recommendations. In the oversight meeting before the sub-committee, Holohan had been on the receiving end of a slap-down from Martin Fraser and the two civil servants found themselves on opposite sides once more. Senior officials took exception to the CMO's and NPHET's media appearances and repeated warnings, which they saw as an attempt to exert pressure on the Government. 'The Government,' Fraser told Holohan, 'will make the decision'. The implication was clear: Not you.

When the time came for the Government to make its deliberations at the Cabinet sub-committee, they broadened the range of advice they would take in. NPHET's voice would be diluted. It was a long night in the Sycamore Room. Tired ministers and officials, both in the room and joining via video link, rubbed their eyes and settled in for the long haul.

Presentations given by Ernst and Young supported the NPHET viewpoint on hospitality, highlighting the raft of new cases that had followed the reopening of wet pubs in September 2020, as well as the impact of the Thanksgiving mixing in Canada on the virus there. The Central Statistics Office showed that the public's overall life satisfaction was multiples worse than it had been in the austerity phase of 2013; the Department of Finance, led by Minister Paschal Donohoe, outlined the huge economic cost of the pandemic and lockdowns to date, running at an eye-watering €1 billion every month.

Paul Reid of the HSE was in the mix too, beaming in from health service headquarters. The message from Reid, as it had been back in October, was that hospitals were coping. As soon as he said it, the NPHET heads dropped. It was a low point in the ongoing cold war between the Department and the HSE. 'This is the Head of our Health Service telling the Government not to worry.' If the muted NPHET microphones were on, they may have picked up one or two deep breaths as Reid reassured the Government that the hospitals were faring well. NPHET members felt betrayed. To their eyes, Reid was kowtowing to the Government while they were going: "Please don't open the pubs. Please don't open the pubs", and Paul's going, "Yeah, well, everything's fine for now, you know, and we've invested in our ICU and we're coping."'

Reid's public stance caused consternation with the HSE too. More than one member of its senior structure was dismayed by the constant reassurance about the hospital network's ability to withstand Christmas. The official says the positions publicly taken by the HSE in the run-up to Christmas were 'frankly wrong'.

'You can't go about reassuring people that we have enough beds. That's reassurance based on not understanding how the disease model forecast rapid escalation of cases,' the person says, adding that if they had been at a press conference alongside Reid in late November or early December, they certainly couldn't, and wouldn't, back up misplaced soothsaying that everything was going to be fine.

Paul Reid, for his part, is open about his misgivings about the NPHET process. He felt October was a mess that caused a great deal of unnecessary tension. It was 'inevitable', though, he felt. 'It was going to burst.' He believes there are times when NPHET has gone too far, perhaps even going over 'the line' public servants shouldn't cross. 'You have to value the Government and democratic process,' he says. 'They are who is elected by the public. The rest of us are there to give them advice.'

He makes a rather dramatic comparison to his old job. Reid, after leaving Eircom, moved to Trócaire. He spent time in Africa, South America and Asia. 'I don't want to go to the extreme but having spent time in developing countries, if you don't value the government process, the democratic process, it's a very different system you live in. I just think over the last year or so, that's how tensions emerge. Whether it's NIAC [the National Immunisation Advisory Committee] or whether it's NPHET. We have to remind ourselves we're not decision makers, you know.'

Reid, linking in to the discussions in the Sycamore Room via video link on a separate line to his NPHET counterparts, continued to hammer home the message that hospitals were secure. In his view, he played it with a 'straight bat'; information from his hospital managers was telling him that things were not much more strained than normal. Despite that, many senior medics across the country, particularly in Dublin, felt they were already under pressure and harboured fears about the Christmas to come.

Another group was also in the mix. The ESRI presented behavioural analysis in advance of the Cabinet sub-committee meeting. The institute had been subject to duelling claims by NPHET and the Department of the Taoiseach, with different findings held by both sides to try to justify their arguments. Researchers felt exposed.

When it came to the big moment on decisions for December, the projections from Philip Nolan came through. Some of the ESRI's researchers were staggered. 'My God,' they muttered to each other. They couldn't believe the Government was pushing ahead with the reopening of hospitality, based on what the projections had said. Collectively, they felt that this was a risk the Government should not take. Their own research showed the public were on the same track too, with a clear majority of people calling for restrictions through December if it meant they could see family and friends in the week around Christmas. However, the public did want to see pubs and restaurants open (with social distancing) rather than staying closed until the New Year.

The Taoiseach was facing a tightrope decision that would define not only his premiership but, more important, the lives of thousands of people across the country. He hesitated. He had sat in his office late at night all week in the run-up to the Cabinet sub-committee meeting and the announcement. His mind was racked with doubt.

His parliamentary party was roaring for pubs to be reopened. Some TDs – Marc MacSharry, Jim O'Callaghan and others – were telling him to ignore NPHET and push Ireland back to Level 2 on the reopening plan. To them, Level 3 would not cut it for thousands of businesses across Ireland.

In the back of Martin's mind was a doubt. One that would cross his mind as he sat in the office, chatting to his staff. 'I'd have preferred a delay of a week at the time,' he says. 'I don't think it would have had a huge impact but I would have preferred a delay.'

Leo Varadkar had doubts, too. Newspapers, radio shows and discussions at parliamentary party meetings had all been framed around the lockdown to 'Save Christmas'. It's a turn of phrase that Varadkar came to loathe, often rolling his eyes unsubtly when he heard it. To his mind, it created a dangerous expectation of normality – that the public could go back to socializing as they had done last Christmas before the pandemic, as if they could close their eyes and wish away Covid and wake up in 2019. 'If you say to people that, you know, you've been through a six-week lockdown, there's now three or four weeks between now and Christmas where you can do all the things you missed out on – and then there's potentially going to be another set of restrictions in January – you're potentially saying to people, here's your opportunity to socialize and to mix,' he says.

Varadkar caused trouble for the Government in the week before the crunch decision. Fianna Fáil TDs and members of Varadkar's own party, not to mention Sinn Féin and the wider public, were incensed by his comments that cross-border travel should be tightened when restrictions eased due to the North's higher Covid rates at the time. He had also told the Dáil in November that people shouldn't be looking to book flights home, comparing the situation to 1967's foot-and-mouth crisis appeal to emigrants to stay away.

NPHET spelled out its position. It recommended that hospitality remain closed, except for takeaway or delivery, for the remainder of the year. It also recommended the public be allowed to visit one other household in the run-up to 21 December; and from that point, three households could be allowed to mix, with households urged to take 'no more than one significant trip' in that timeframe.

Their modelling showed a worst-case scenario of 1,500 cases per day in late January, based on what might be expected with hospitality and household visits combined. NPHET suggested that if cases passed a threshold of 400, and if thereafter there was exponential growth, the Government should step in with a short, sharp three-week shutdown. This would give Professor Philip Nolan and his modelling colleagues a reproduction rate (R number) for the virus of 1.4–1.6. The calculation was vastly underestimated.

Members of the Government point to the fact that the NPHET modelling showed that, with household visits continuing and hospitality closed, an R number of 1.1–1.2 was the likely scenario. The gap between the two scenarios may seem small, but in the model presented at their briefing it would be the difference between 300 to 500 cases per day in mid- to late January (R1.1 and R1.2) and between three and five times as many – up to 1,500 (R1.4 and R1.6).

Minister Eamon Ryan's view was that 'the overall assessment on a modelling basis was much of a muchness. There wasn't a huge element of difference.' For Leo Varadkar, the decision not to heed the NPHET modelling was 'partly' because of NPHET's 'overreaction' back in October and, in Varadkar's view, before. 'We'd several instances now where they had kind of predicted doom and it hadn't materialized. This time they didn't predict doom.'

Doom was on the minds of NPHET's members, however. Dr Mary Favier says there is an element of truth in Varadkar's words. 'There is an element of when you're in NPHET, you're in this little echo chamber of anxiety and worry that it'll all go south again. It does make us cautious. But before Christmas, all the signs were that this was going to go bad.' The Varadkar targeting of NPHET and Holohan back in October? That 'didn't help by any means,' she says.

Holohan's letter and presentation warned that if the Government did go against their advice and reopen hospitality, there could be no extension of household visits beyond one home over Christmas. Angrily, one NPHET member shakes their head and says, the weight of what was to come etched on their face, 'It wasn't presented as a choice, and if it was, why the fuck would you pick pubs over families being allowed to meet up?'

'We thought this [allowing household visits] was an important measure,' says another key member of NPHET. 'It's been such a difficult year for people. People have been locked away for so long that it might help in terms of mental health and all other considerations. We thought locking people away and stopping people from meeting up completely was very draconian. It was very draconian and we didn't want to continue it. This wasn't a choice.'

Minister Paschal Donohoe saw the weight of the decision everywhere he went. As he turned down a deserted Dawson Street, a man came up to him and burst out crying in front of him, tears running down his face. He had had to close his business, his pride and joy. It happened again on Pembroke Street; a man outside a restaurant caught sight of the Finance Minister and let fly with a volley of roars. As he continued to shout, he became emotional and upset.

'We get the emails and the letters,' Donohoe says, 'but you just saw it in people coming up to you, you saw it in their eyes. It is true that NPHET wanted us to go at a far slower pace than we did.' For him, however, the impact of six long weeks of lockdown after a year of misery needed to be lifted. A tired public, he felt, couldn't take any more.

On Friday, 27 November, the Cabinet would meet to reopen the country. It may have been shaping up to be a Christmas unlike any other, but some traditions would never change and they became obstacles. The meeting wasn't the only show in town that day. It was also the date of the *Late Late Toy Show*. Politicians and officials scrambled in the week running up to the announcement trying to figure out a timeframe so that Micheál Martin wasn't standing at a podium 'pissing people off' while the most-watched television programme of the year was forced to take a back seat. 'We'll be slaughtered,' said one minister in a WhatsApp message to me the week before, adding that if the Government had any sense they'd get everything done by the Thursday to avoid the clash.

Word had leaked from the Cabinet sub-committee the night before and the hospitality industry largely welcomed the reopening, bar vintners, who raised what they deemed the unequal treatment of wet pubs.

Standing outside Government Buildings on the Friday wasn't an ideal backdrop for broadcasting. The rain poured in buckets, drenching through trouser legs and into socks. Noel Anderson, the amiable and media-friendly chair of the Licensed Vintners Association, battled with his brolly in the gusts at the Virgin Media News live point as ministers came and went from what was a rubber-stamp exercise on the decisions made the night before.

Two ministers, one of them involved in the Cabinet sub-committee, stopped by to ask had I anywhere booked for a meal. Having spent months waiting to get out of Dublin and safely down to my partner in West Cork, the thought of going for a meal wasn't a priority for me personally. I told them I was going to wait until after Christmas Day. This was met with raised eyebrows and a sceptical 'oh right' as they spelled out what they had lined up for the days and weeks ahead. Like so many others, they were looking forward to the chance to meet up once again with friends and treat family members they'd been locked away from to a night away from the pandemic.

Ministers were optimistic. 'We've done it' was their confident message. There were sore feelings about the plight of 'wet pubs', again told they would not be reopening due to the risk of super-spreading, but there was an undercurrent of excitement that the worst of the pandemic was being left in the rear view mirror on Merrion Street. 'This will all be over by next summer,' said one Fianna Fáil minister. 'We won't even be talking about it. You'll have to find something else to report on.'

The unlocking confirmation was warmly welcomed across politics. Sinn Féin's Mary Lou McDonald welcomed the 'clarity' given by the Government, saying they had to 'strike a balance and I think that's what they've sought to do'. Columnists praised the Government for 'exerting its authority' over NPHET, with hundreds of cases per day marked as a 'price worth paying'; others said it was a 'major risk' to open the country despite warnings from medics but a 'most welcome development' for most of the country.

As the Taoiseach took the podium, after a rehearsal and mic-check minutes before, blinking in the spotlight that was a touch too bright, he once again leaned on an expression that had previously been leaned on in the days of late November – this would be a 'meaningful Christmas', one where people would take personal responsibility, with every contact counting.

Tony Holohan and his colleagues had been left out of the political circle for the announcement. Their appearances at lockdown easing announcements had fallen off considerably over time. Holohan was immediately concerned by the plan. 'I was very worried,' he says. 'I really was of the view that this would increase socialization very significantly and create the opportunity for super-spreading events.'

There was more than a note of despair among the medics. 'No fucking question in my mind about it, I think we're fucked,' was the instant reaction of one NPHET member. 'What the fuck are we doing?'

Holohan and co. knew bad times were ahead. What they didn't know was that moving to Level 3 would prompt a rise of socializing to pre-pandemic levels. They didn't predict Ireland's infection rate surging to become the highest anywhere in the world. They didn't foretell the arrival of a new variant of the virus that would pour petrol on a bonfire that would consume the country.

The relationship between Ireland's Government and its key health advisers entered the most critical moment of the pandemic battered and bruised. A rupture had been exposed just weeks earlier, on that one weekend in October, when the virus was relegated to second rung on the ladder of hostilities. High-ranking members of the Cabinet accused NPHET of unrealistic expectations, of having tried to 'usurp' their power and, crucially, of overstepping and ignoring their diplomatic mandate. For their part, many NPHET members believe that the Government had played fast and loose with the health of the nation and had fuelled an atmosphere where they, mere advisers, had become the human shield for the Government after months of frustration and fatigue.

The Christmas and New Year period to come would see tens of thousands of people infected with coronavirus. Nurses and doctors in hospitals were pushed to breaking point, watching many of their colleagues fall ill, forced to decide whether or not critical care could be offered to patients as ICUs swelled to capacity and beyond. Many hundreds of lives were lost in villages and towns across Ireland, with the sorrow of loss to this day still not processed by the mourners who lined the streets to say farewell to too many neighbours, too many fathers, mothers, sons and daughters.

The following weeks would be the darkest of a State in emergency.

Chapter 15: The Board

Department of Public Health Mid-West,
Limerick, 24 December 2020

Everyone remembers the board.

At face value, there is nothing unique about it. It's a regular-sized whiteboard – taller than it is wide, scrawled letters and numbers dotted across it in marker pen on top of untidy smears where yesterday's figures were wiped away. The office of the Department of Public Health Mid-West, at the corner of Mount Kennett Place and Henry Street in Limerick City, is entirely unremarkable. You would forget it was there. In fact, people did. At the outset, when Feed the Heroes was sending much-needed supplies and food to hospitals, fire stations and Gardaí across the country, they were passed by. Nobody knew that a team of highly specialized doctors and nurses were at war, the sentries clearing Covid from bunkers in schools, factories and nursing homes.

That thoroughly unremarkable board, which sits against the back wall, visible from all corners of the open-plan office, shows the locations and number of cases and outbreaks right across the Mid-West, from Limerick, Clare and North Tipperary. On Christmas Eve, it lit up in green and red felt-tip pen; festive colours, but this was no cause for celebration. The phones rang and rang. Surveillance staff added even more numbers to the board. 'Outbreak, nursing home, five confirmed cases, one death.'

What the rapidly filling whiteboard told was the story of a tragedy escalating at a disturbing rate. The third wave had started to roar. The public health team in the Mid-West was witnessing it crash ashore in real time. 'It was like a visualized tsunami coming at you,' says public health nurse Maura Richardson. The board named nursing homes, the number of cases and, tragically, the number of deaths. Unlike most natural disasters, the team had known that this was on the way. The case numbers from early December, to their mind, were too high.

Regional public health teams are unique and yet, still, to many within the speciality, their work remains unheralded. In truth, public health teams in a pandemic are Covid detectives. They follow leads on outbreaks at weddings, in nursing homes, in restaurants, and they will begin work to investigate where they came from and who else might be infected. It's a combination of surveillance and management, rooting out the virus and stopping it in its tracks, preventing it spreading to more households or vulnerable groups like people in nursing homes.

Its head of department is Dr Mai Mannix. The best way to understand it, she believes, is to look at it as 'like being a helicopter overseeing your whole population. You know exactly where the cases are. You know the names of everybody. You know everybody who dies, sadly. You kind of follow the ones that come across your desk, the ones that end up going to ICU and you root for them. "Please keep going." And then you see when they pass on. It's terrible.'

From the very first day of the pandemic in the Mid-West, the team were up against it, she says. One of the first cases in the country was on their patch, with hundreds of contacts sprawling across schools and workplaces.

The focus for the team in the early days was round-the-clock contact tracing. There were no national call centres for contact tracing; all that work was done by the regional teams. Testing was limited and needed to be protected. The public health teams were the gatekeepers for all swab requests, making sure they were being used appropriately. That required extreme vigilance. The phone would ring at three or four in the morning, not that anyone was sleeping much at that time anyway. Dr Marie Casey, one of the four specialists working alongside Mai, would handle calls from the National Ambulance Service from her bed in the middle of the night and then get up and arrive at the office by 8 a.m. to start a full day's work.

Just sixteen people staffed the department from the outset. It couldn't last. Reinforcements were drafted in from all corners. They came from across the HSE, and from non-medical sectors of the public service: staff were called up from the Department of Education, from Limerick Institute of Technology and from Limerick City and County Council. This was a conscription-style deployment. One of the members who was drafted to a regional public health team likens the situation to the misfits cobbled together for the Home Guard in *Dad's Army,* though that would be an unfair comparison to make considering the speed at which people had to adapt to their new roles as tracers.

As the first wave rocked the Mid-West, it was immediately clear that nursing homes were at the epicentre. Dr Rose Fitzgerald led the department's response. Fitzgerald was the most seasoned investigator on the team, with more than twenty years in the department working on infectious diseases. And yet 'nothing could have prepared anybody' for what was happening, she says. 'Our parents and grandparents had world wars. This is what war is for us.'

She will always remember that first nursing home. People began to get sick without known contact with Covid. By the time testers were deployed, there was already too much infection among very ill residents and staff who may have been asymptomatic. A call would come in from a nursing home alerting her to a case among residents. The first stop for the public health doctors is a risk assessment – trying to figure out if the outbreak can deteriorate or if it's already worse than it first appeared. It almost always was.

Doctors Fitzgerald, Casey and their colleagues would then run through a checklist: 'Okay, can that staff member isolate? Can we move everyone who is suspected Covid away from non-Covid? Have you got enough PPE?' That final question was as protracted an issue in the Mid-West as anywhere else. Such was the concern that Dr Casey went to the dusty storeroom in the department and found every last mask, glove and goggle she could, stuffing them in a cardboard box and sticking it in a taxi to go across Limerick to the Community Health Organisation to use across nursing homes.

The horror drove some nursing home staff they contacted past their limit. In some instances, staff quit on the spot and didn't come back. 'They just walked,' says Rose. 'Just said "I'm not going to work any more."' Marie saw it happen too. 'An awful lot of people refused to go back to work after they were excluded [by positive test or close contact]. They just said: "I'm not going back. I can't face that again."'

In some homes with severe outbreaks, some nursing staff resigned. 'They might have been the only staff member left who was clear to work,' says Marie. From the office in the city centre, Rose and Marie contacted nurses who could be working two days and two nights in a row, battling to protect their residents at a time when even the most basic care became a challenge.

It is a harrowing thing for any healthcare worker to see. Vulnerable residents, Covid patients, left behind in their moment of need.

Some of their colleagues volunteered to step in to fill that gap they were shaken to see open. Doctors from other areas of medicine volunteered to take on duties reserved for HCAs and nurses. They fed people, minded them, helped them to the toilet.

The pressure to volunteer extended even to nurses working in the public health team. Nurse Bernie Higgins had completed a twelve-hour shift in the department and was 'dog tired' from the unending workload. The phone rang as she was clocking out. 'Could you possibly do a night shift for us?' Another nursing home was crumbling under the virus's power. She was stunned. Stopping in her tracks, she grabbed her phone straight from her pocket and called her sister. 'Will I do it? Should I do it?' she asked. 'We all felt guilty that we weren't doing enough,' Bernie says. It was 'traumatic'.

The trauma and stress were felt right across the department. Rose Fitzgerald would wake in the middle of the night worrying about the outbreaks she had dealt with in the office. 'What's going on in that nursing home?'; 'What can we do about that outbreak?' Her brain could not switch off. This was a twenty-four-hour job.

'Lots and lots and lots of people died,' she says. Anywhere between a quarter and a fifth of residents who became infected in major nursing home outbreaks could lose their lives. There were instances across the region where eight residents died, ten residents died, twelve residents died. Sometimes even more. Public health nurse Rachel Brickenden says, 'We had forty nursing homes up on that board. There were double-digit cases and double-digit deaths.'

The tide of the pandemic receded in the summer months but there was no end to the work. The reopening of bars and restaurants just shifted the hunt for the virus to a new arena. Outbreaks were traced to people spending hours in the pub, infecting not just their own group, but others nearby. The virus would be transmitted from one group of six to the next group of six at the table nearest to them. Sometimes, as many as twenty cases would be linked to these incidents.

The contact tracing regime for restaurants and pubs, where customers in a group would leave one name and mobile phone number at the business, meant awkward conversations for the public health staff to try to get the names and numbers of everyone who had been there. It was tiresome work. Sometimes, the team would go back and check CCTV to see who was near index cases and what tables were at risk. Some restaurants were 'devastated' by the news that there had been outbreaks. 'Many felt responsible, in some way,' says Mai Mannix. But it wasn't their fault. They followed the guidelines on table spacing, how long customers could stay, and on contact tracing. It just wasn't enough. Risk was everywhere. Covid reached far beyond two metres of distance.

Some of the extra bodies brought in to handle the first wave returned to their regular jobs, their own duties calling them away. The permanent staff and those who stayed were left feeling abandoned, short on staff and low on resources for a job they knew was far from finished. They were still working with obsolete software. They were working through exhaustion. At the peak of the first wave, the numbers had swollen to sixty people. They gradually ebbed away as the immediate threat dropped.

In August 2020, Marie Casey sat at her computer until 11 p.m., typing out page after page and document after document. The 'old ways' of bureaucracy meant that if the department wanted more staff, it would need to issue business cases to justify each member brought in for the coming wave of the virus. These were seven-page documents and they were drawn up for multiple individual requests for temporary cover. Often they disappeared into the ether. The department's early SOS signals went unanswered.

A handful of reinforcements joined the fold. One of them was Eamonn Franklin, of Limerick City and County Council's Housing Assistance Payment scheme. He had spotted an email from the HSE looking for volunteers and mulled it over that summer. An analytical man, he weighed up the pros and cons. He felt it wouldn't look bad on the CV in years to come and the fact that it looked like fairly straightforward administrative work was a plus, giving him more time to spend at home with his wife and two kids than his regular job would. He arrived in November for a three-month exchange and put himself about, looking to help in whatever way he could. He was still there eight months later, fully immersed in the team.

In the midst of it all, Eamonn's sense of humour became something of a boon for the department. A tall, bald man in an office almost exclusively staffed by women, he would sense when people needed a lift and put himself out there to take a slagging. 'Bad hair day,' he'd mutter to one of the women in the office, who he knew would be game for a laugh. Her response would set others off who had been working away quietly. Before you'd know it, everyone would be rowing in with their two cents to have a cut off Eamonn.

The chemistry of the team is very evident around the floor. If a contact tracer is struggling to make a link between cases, someone like Eamonn, who has a good memory for names, will step in and help to join the dots. Nurses, surveillance staff, registrars all knock on Mai's or Marie's or Rose's door with queries. It's a collaborative effort and when the staff there say they've never exchanged cross words with each other or stormed out in a huff even on the toughest days, you believe them. That camaraderie would be needed in the months ahead.

By the time winter came around, the threadbare public health team knew what was coming. As the Taoiseach took to the podium to announce the loosening of restrictions for a 'meaningful Christmas', there was sorrow in the meeting room. They had been through this before. Now, armed with the traumatic memories of the first surge, they felt the country was being led into danger. One doctor threw her notebook on the floor. 'That was it. We knew,' says Dr Casey. 'We knew the case numbers were too high when they opened up to keep in any way manageable.'

Dr Mannix anxiously surveyed her team. 'I think we knew in our hearts we were in for a hammering.' As a leader, she is universally respected; she's known to go around thanking people individually for their efforts on any given day. Everyone in the department looked up to her, feeling appreciated, no matter what task they were on. Mannix sorely wanted them all to have a break at Christmas to spend time with their families, revelling in the joy and laughter of their small children, and recharge for whatever lay in wait in the New Year. In her heart, she knew this hope was dashed.

'We knew it was coming, we really did,' she says. 'There's nothing you can do.' Even before Christmas, the volume of calls and cases were on the up. Casey and Fitzgerald had already been forced to consult the framework about how to prioritize outbreaks. Some would get attention. Others would not. 'Things just didn't get done,' says Fitzgerald. Casey puts it plainly: 'We had to leave outbreaks in certain settings and just let them go and not investigate them. We just didn't have the capacity.'

Then it came. The whiteboard had remained a constant throughout the pandemic, but on Christmas Eve it became something else entirely. People remember the sound of phones constantly ringing; colleagues walking back and forth from the board, marking up new cases in a named nursing home, or outbreaks linked to a workplace or household visit. It did not let up.

Rose Fitzgerald was standing in as Acting Director of Public Health that Christmas Eve. That evening, she sent an email up the line. It was a clear message, effectively a distress call, that the infrastructure around public health had buckled under the weight of infections. They were overrun. 'What we have now, we simply cannot follow up.'

Specialist registrar Dr Mark O'Loughlin had joined the team in the Mid-West after the first wave. He was on duty that Christmas Eve and for St Stephen's Day. Something wasn't adding up. He was reading the news reports of the cases announced nationally by NPHET. They weren't tallying with what he was seeing coming through on the board. There were torrents of information and they wouldn't stop coming. The decades-old CIDR (Computerised Infectious Disease Reporting) software folded. 'It couldn't cope with the numbers,' he says, adding damningly, 'which was hardly surprising given its age.' He was no stranger to these issues. In his previous workplace, he remembers, 'They had to get programmers out of retirement to keep the system running. That's what we were dealing with.'

Mark tapped away at admin work at home for hours that night and many others. He would remotely access the HSE network and stay up until 3 a.m., just to get basic administrative work out of the way. He stayed working through to the small hours just so he could focus on the clinical work the next day. 'This is not normal,' he told himself time after time. 'If I worked anywhere else in the world, I wouldn't have to do this.'

Mai Mannix knew what was happening and knew it wouldn't be limited to the Mid-West. She kept the HSE informed, phoning Dr Lorraine Doherty, the HSE's National Clinical Director for Health Protection; Dr Kevin Kelleher, the Assistant National Director for Public Health, who was also based in the Limerick office; and Dr John Cuddihy of the HPSC. She was telling them that the Mid-West was in 'real trouble' and pleading for immediate help. At that point, it was all she could do. 'The whole thing was collapsing around our ears,' she says. 'It's your worst nightmare. It was horrendous. My staff worked fourteen- to sixteen-hour days over Christmas and New Year, coming in extra days, over weekends, everything.' The pressure wouldn't lift for weeks, pushing staff to the very brink.

The third wave devastated nursing homes in the region. Eight residents had died at a home in Newcastle West by 4 January. Twenty died in Caherconlish. In Cahercalla in County Clare, the Defence Forces were called in to assist during a major outbreak that saw twenty-three residents and twenty-three staff infected.

'There was constant pressure. We had this feeling of this wall of cases and the deaths were horrendous,' says Marie Casey. Even getting through to the homes was a major challenge. 'The staff were overwhelmed, they couldn't pick up the phone. You had to really struggle to find out what was going on.' Mark O'Loughlin says it was 'like watching thirty people try to build a big jigsaw puzzle collaboratively. All of us were just trying to pitch in here and there, ducking and diving between "what is this crisis?", "what is the next crisis?"' Everyone felt the exhaustion.

Marie Casey suffered on those days. 'The deaths killed me,' she says. The team would meet at nine o'clock for the morning meeting. The scale of loss and the speed at which it was ripping through care settings was immeasurable. It did not seem to end. A decision was taken. 'We stopped having the death total on the board,' says Marie. A staff member scrubbed it off. It didn't go back up. 'Part of me thinks it's because we couldn't keep track. The other part of me thinks it's because we couldn't look at it any more.'

More people died in the Mid-West in January and February 2021 than died in all of 2020. In the nursing homes, it came with a cruel twist, killing residents who were mere days or weeks from vaccination. 'They were so close. They were just there. Just a few more weeks if we'd …'

She stops. This was the first time Marie has cried since the start of the pandemic. The first time she's had a single moment to process what was happening – at a loss for words to try to encapsulate the pain. 'Sometimes, I'd see a case and I'd look them up on RIP.ie just to see a picture. Just to know them.'

Marie is clear in her view on the third wave. 'We could have prevented this. If we'd waited a few more weeks, we could have saved these people.' The public, she says, were not to blame for the surge. 'People did what they were told was okay. People were told they could visit restaurants, could go to the pub in groups and believed they would be safe.'

The emotional toll of grief for people who they never met but cared for and battled so hard to protect, coupled with the physical exhaustion, took many to a state of burnout. For Mark O'Loughlin, how will he look back on all of this, when it's all over and he's years removed from this period of relentless stress; what will his memories be of the Covid-19 pandemic from his public health perspective? His answer is deadpan. 'I don't think I slept enough to be able to form memories.'

The public health nurses feel the public will never quite understand the sorrow of January 2021. Maura Richardson says that despite the headlines, the constant media coverage and the return to a full Level 5 lockdown, the public 'saw what they wanted to see'.

Tackling the spread in the general population was a minefield too. Contact tracing calls were harder over Christmas. Sometimes the nurses would be abused and shouted at down the phone. At one point, it seemed as if people just stopped answering their phones altogether. Many didn't show for their Covid tests either. Data compiled by the department at the end of 2020 showed that 960 people in Limerick, Clare and North Tipperary failed to appear for their scheduled test appointment over the Christmas period.

'I thought I was safe,' one Covid patient told Marie Casey on the phone. They had gone out for dinner with friends and gone back to work in a nursing home. Eighty people were infected with Covid. 'These are not bad people. They were just doing ordinary human things that they were told were okay to do.'

The Mid-West department pulled itself through because nobody else would. All the way through the pandemic they have focused on their patients – all 397,000 people across the region – and deep down, their thoughts were about trying to keep as many of them alive as possible.

To keep the region safe, they put their lives on hold. 'It came at huge personal cost,' says Mai Mannix. 'Little ones haven't seen their mums or dads for a number of weeks and then they go home and the little ones are just so upset.' Marie Casey battled burnout from early in the year. She had come back from maternity leave just before the pandemic, following the birth of her son. 'He was crying all night because I wasn't around,' she says. 'He had a mom who was around for ages before that. A lot of my colleagues' kids were very distressed.' She hit a wall early on in the pandemic. Bouncing between home, sleepless nights, the office and the deluge of new cases and crises week after week. 'I just kept thinking about patients all of the time and worrying about what was going to happen next. Worrying about cases and cases and cases. Normally, I'm really good at compartmentalizing, but this time there was no escape.'

At the start of the pandemic, Ireland had fewer senior public health doctors like Mai Mannix, Rose Fitzgerald, Marie Casey, Breda Cosgrove and Anne Dee than comparable countries. We had sixty. Scotland had 179. New Zealand had 169. All of those doctors in Scotland and New Zealand were employed at consultant level. In Ireland, they were not. For twenty years, the public health specialists of Ireland, more than eighty per cent of whom are women, fought for consultant contracts, parity of esteem and parity of pay with the rest of their colleagues across Irish medicine.

Multiple reports pointed to failings in surveillance software, staffing shortages and an ageing workforce long before the arrival of Covid. In 2014, the Royal College of Physicians Ireland warned that Ireland would urgently need to boost specialist numbers because of 'the lack of a universal primary health care structure and a less well-developed public health service to deal with emergencies (e.g. pandemic flu)'.

The public health teams battled through the first, second and third waves without any recourse to industrial relations, deferring a planned strike before Christmas on ethical grounds due to the rapidly deteriorating situation. In April 2021, it was finally announced by the Health Minister Stephen Donnelly that consultant contracts would be open to public health doctors. On Friday, 7 May, that deal was ratified, by eighty-seven per cent, by the Irish Medical Organisation's public health doctors. It was a huge relief and could mark the beginning of a change that is long overdue.

The trauma of Covid will be carried with them for ever. But they can stand proud. At Christmas, Mai gathered the staff together and addressed them. Whatever the numbers were in the community, in that darkest hour, she said, it would have been triple that if it weren't for the work that was done within that building. It was a speech that steeled a lot of the staff there to get through the worst moment of their professional lives.

'I am extremely proud,' says Mai. 'They have gone over and above every single time.' Without that thankless work on what became known as the forgotten frontline, she has no doubt that many more lives would have been lost.

Chapter 16: The Fear

Belmullet, County Mayo, January 2021

Sean Conroy will remember it for the rest of his life. As the hearse turned left to head for the funeral home, the ambulance behind turned right on the long road to Castlebar hospital. 'He missed his wife's funeral,' Conroy remembers, a pallor coming over his face. 'He had to watch it on an iPad in a hospital bed.' Ambulances were a regular sight in Belmullet that dark January of 2021. So were hearses.

Conroy, a funeral director and school principal in the town, would see his own father make the same journeys. And, were it not for some luck, he could have too. At least twelve Covid funerals took place in the Erris area over the course of the month. Belmullet, a town of around two thousand people on the north-west coast of Mayo, was the focal point of a surge of infections in the local electoral area (LEA), which became a centre of attention for Ireland's third wave.

Belmullet was a magnet for headlines both at home and abroad. At its peak, according to official figures, one in seventeen people in the LEA contracted the virus over a two-week period – more than four times the national average. Some local medics believe the figure is likely an underestimate. Other parts of Erris and the Mullet peninsula, an area the size of County Louth, were less affected than others. In the more populated parts of the region, the true figure could have been as high as one in ten over the period.

While the news focused on the surge in infections, an online blame game erupted. Many businesses and individuals were singled out and accused of breaches that caused the surge. Locals feel the personal tragedy of the region was lost in the clamour in the national press and in anonymous whisperings online. Comment after comment, tweet after tweet, pointing the finger of blame at businesses as people tried to find something, *anything* to channel their anger towards.

In a torrid winter of gales and storms, the people of Erris stood out on windy hills overlooking the Atlantic, hoods up, rain battering their faces, to say farewell to neighbours, friends, colleagues and loved ones who were taken from them by coronavirus. 'We were absolutely torn asunder,' says a local businessman. 'There hasn't been a family that doesn't know someone lost to this virus.'

The surge began in the run-up to Christmas. The Mayo footballers, a unique unifying force in the county's identity, were once again togging out to play in the All-Ireland Football Final against Dublin under the bright lights at an empty Croke Park, hosting its first December final since 1917. The usual 'Mayo for Sam' excitement lit up the gloomy weeks of the November lockdown. 'Can they do it?'; 'Will they do it?' People, as they always do, came together to watch the match. Some returned home a week early for Christmas to be there for it. There were house parties. There were people who came back from Dublin or England or further afield to be a part of the excitement and to stay on for Christmas.

The impact was instant.

On 28 December, Dr Fergal Ruane was the lone GP on call for Erris. Bank holiday Mondays are always busy mornings on the phones. Rubbing his eyes and getting set for the day ahead, he told his wife, Maria – who also worked in the practice – that it might start getting busy at 11 a.m., anticipating a build-up of the usual bumps, bruises and illnesses that might have arisen over the weekend, nothing to do with Covid. By ten o'clock, he'd called her over. The switchboard screen flashed with blinking lights.

Both of them were on the phone right up to 8 p.m. that night without leaving the surgery. It was call after call. 'Is there anyone else in the house? What symptoms do they have?' Fergal had suspected that post-Christmas would be bad – 'I think the Government went too, "Ah, we're grand now and everything will be fine" and I think that led to some people being complacent' – but he could never have imagined this.

Complacency, he says, couldn't have been the only factor. People in the area were careful, including the most vulnerable in the town. One older woman, he says, who he met for vaccination the following month, hadn't left her house in a year, shutting herself off from the world to protect herself from the invisible threat. 'The one time she went was to the beach when she knew there'd be nobody there. Other than that, the only other people she saw were the guys delivering her groceries.'

The virus ran riot. The GPs and their surgery teams were referring over one hundred people per day for testing, including whole families. For people working at the swabbing centres, sometimes you could tell a whole car was sick by looking in the windows at the white faces and the shattered demeanour, with small babies often screaming crying in the back seat. This was the most explosive impact of Covid any village in Ireland had yet to see. Dozens were treated in Mayo University Hospital in Castlebar, in Galway University Hospital and in the Community Hospital in Belmullet. Local health teams were run ragged; they had never been busier. It is unlikely they ever will be again.

Dr Ruane himself was infected with Covid, having to continue work over the telephone because he was unable to secure a locum to cover. Fergal's symptoms were debilitating. He would take one or two phone calls and then, struggling to speak through exhaustion, have to pause with fatigue. 'I spent three or four days where I don't think I've ever been as sick as that in my life. You're obviously worried because you knew that with a volume of cases like this, there was going to be a death toll, for want of a better word.'

'Within two days of Christmas,' says Fr Kevin Hegarty, of neighbouring Kilmore Erris parish, who lives in Belmullet, 'Christmas was over here. People had begun to go down with Covid, even younger people.'

By mid-January, more than thirty people in the area had been referred to hospital, several of them to intensive care. Around Belmullet, the psychological impact was haunting. If you stood on the main street, you'd hear no cars, none of the usual chance Christmas meetings or laughter in the street. None of the invitations to meet up for a drink later or to come over with the family. 'It was dystopian,' says Fr Hegarty. Shoppers quickly shuffled through the aisles as they got their bread and milk, getting in and out without engaging with others. By three in the afternoon, the streets were all but bare. The silence, the desolation, was eerie and would continue for weeks to come.

'The community was menaced by this insidious virus,' Fr Hegarty says. 'The fear was, who is going to get hit next?'

* * * *

Paschal Donohoe pored over his notes. Frantically, he pulled them out wherever he could find them. Pages and pages of notes. Every discussion document, every modelling scenario, every Cabinet paper, anything and everything he could find from before Christmas. He had a simple question. 'How did I get it so wrong?'

The alarm had been raised with the Government before Christmas. Cases were rocketing. And a new enemy had revealed itself.

'Stop everything now. Pull the flights.' Eamon Ryan's Junior Minister Ossian Smyth was adamant, the panic of his plea on the phone catching Ryan off-guard. Smyth had been following the developments of a new variant first identified in Kent. The UK Health Secretary, Matt Hancock, had said that this new strain of Covid was 'out of control' in London and the south of England. It was a threat that had been growing and growing. Scientists weren't sure whether its spread was down to it hitting major urban centres at the right time, or if it was, by virtue of its own mutations, more transmissible.

Tier Four restrictions were immediately imposed in London and its surrounds to try to slow down the variant. It was described by Hancock as 'an incredibly difficult end to frankly an awful year'. It may have been the end to the year, but the variant, which would in time become known as Alpha, was only just getting started.

Ireland, on 20 December, immediately cancelled all flights for forty-eight hours. 'In the interests of public health, people in Britain, regardless of nationality, should not travel to Ireland by air or sea.' The impact was brutal. Thousands of families, separated for a year or more, keeping in touch through stilted Zoom chats, watching grandchildren grow through the lens of a smartphone camera, were denied their Christmas together. Many others travelled anyway, stopping in Belfast on their way home.

The variant was one thing. The transmission at home was another. On the same day, Tony Holohan posted a tweet: 'Cases rising quickly. We have low cases and deaths compared to EU/UK/US. This is at risk now – just as vaccines arrive. To protect yourself & those you love: Stay home. Don't meet up. Stay away from restaurants/pubs. Avoid crowds. Use masks. Follow health advice.'

He was instantly criticized by the hospitality sector. Restaurants Association of Ireland CEO Adrian Cummins said Holohan was stepping 'beyond the line' and urged the Government to reprimand him. Others in Fianna Fáil and Fine Gael were furious too. Marc MacSharry, by now a regular critic of the lockdown policies, suggested it was a 'red herring' to point to pubs and restaurants as problematic. The writing was on the wall, however, and ministers were spooked. In off-the-record comments to media, some put the blame on too many people socializing.

Tony Holohan's view was clear. 'The country because of the package of measures went fully back to normal and behaved as if the pandemic was not there.' It was party time for much of the country. A casual scroll through Instagram on any weekday or weekend night through early December would show you packed pubs and restaurants as people tried to cast off the shackles of the virus with a €9 meal with friends and make sure a year to forget really was forgotten. 'The level of compliance was very, very poor then,' says Holohan. 'I think people saw a decision to allow pubs to be open as essentially a green light to say: 'Well look, if the pub is open, how could this other thing be dangerous?' We couldn't have created better conditions for what happened over the course of that Christmas and January.'

Health Minister Stephen Donnelly was briefed on 17 December on the rapid deterioration. It was a sobering encounter. The number of close contacts being reported per confirmed case had pushed up to an average of 3.6. On the same day, NPHET spelled it out. Holohan said we were in the early stages of a third wave of infection, with the timing of surge in cases 'clearly related to the change' in measures on 4 December. Days later, on the twenty-second, the Taoiseach was forced to close pubs and restaurants from 3 p.m. on Christmas Eve. The shutters would be coming down early.

Paschal Donohoe continued to rummage through the sheets

of paper scattered across his desk in the Department of Finance, overlooked by his family photos and a collection of Star Wars and X-Men bobbleheads: 'Where did I get it wrong?'

'What was so difficult,' he says, 'is you realize that you made a decision and it was a factor in the disease flaring up again. It is true that NPHET wanted us to go at a far slower pace than we did, but you know, I was seeing the effect of this in the eyes of people, in their mental health. I can see it in myself.' Donohoe says that, bar speaking with his family, he has never reflected on the moment or spoken about this burden with anyone publicly. The weight is clear. He leans back in the seat in the same office in the Department of Finance with his hands on his head and his mind goes back to the days before Christmas when the peril of what was to come was laid bare. 'I'm not saying the decisions we made were the sole cause of it – there was the variant question, the household contact was far higher than we were asking it to be in the guidance … I had to say that [our decisions] were part of the cause of it, because they were.'

The day would come for unpacking the decisions and the factors that had led to this deepening emergency. But the focus, for now, had to be on preparing for a wave that was about to do more damage than any one official or politician could have projected or imagined.

Western Road, Cork, December 2020

'And where are you now? … What? … You're in school?' Dr Mary Favier, in her role as GP, was taking calls from her patients. When she fielded a call from a teacher looking for a Covid test while she was at work, she knew Christmas was going to be nightmarish.

More and more patients with symptoms were calling her.

They were not self-isolating. Dr Favier could hear the distinctive ping-ping of supermarket checkout scanners bleeping in the background. Others called from busy platforms at train stations, with the sputtering Tannoy loudly calling out the stops on the journey ahead. Even face to face, patients arriving in her surgery on the northside of Cork City presented with tummy bugs or physical injuries. Only when they were sitting across from her did they also happen to mention, 'while I'm here', that they had been suffering with a ticklish cough for a couple of days, and perhaps mention that their sibling or some other family member had been diagnosed with Covid. 'We had the most extraordinary catalogue of "Really, how could you have missed this?",' she says. 'Christmas and all its baggage was just ourselves as a community doing our thing.'

Other GPs across the country were feeling it too from mid-December. Dr Amy Morgan in Drogheda, County Louth, said she knew it was coming. Everything was up and running as usual in the practice. Childhood vaccinations were going ahead. People were coming in for smear tests. There was a sense of relaxation in the air. People were ready for a Christmas break. The calls with coughs and fevers started to trickle in. Some of Amy's patients, coming back to the family in Drogheda from abroad pre-Christmas, were clearly symptomatic and not keen on isolating. 'You were engaging in a bit of bartering,' she says, '"I think you need a test." And they'd say, "No, no, I don't think so. It's just a winter cold." But you just do not know that.'

The calls kept coming as Christmas week approached. Drogheda was busy. People were going out. 'People had relaxed, you could see it.' Whole households were already infected. Dr Morgan might be dealing with one person on the phone while the rest of the family were in the room and equally in need of tests and isolation advice.

The worst was yet to come.

Cork University Hospital, 19 January 2021

In the Covid ward of CUH, Professor Mary Horgan mopped the sweat off her brow after doffing her PPE. She asked aloud: 'Oh my God, will the numbers coming in ever stop?' The Covid ward was absolutely full and had been since the start of the month. 'You didn't see an end to all of it,' she says. There was no light at the end of the tunnel for staff in the middle of it, or for the patients and their families who were stuck with the most agonising worries.

Professor Horgan was visible and in command. Her distinctive directions echoed through the thirty-five-bed Covid ward as she walked through. She was ever present, an admiral on the deck of a ship that was being swallowed by a tempest. It had become 'a pressure cooker', in the words of Nora Twomey, the Assistant Director of Nursing. Staff point to the visible leadership Horgan showed. If she's here, then we can do this. 'We're together a long time,' says Twomey, 'we have a very strong team around us.' The big concern was staffing. Nora Twomey would think to herself, running through the numbers, 'Do we have enough to do it all again tomorrow?' Often, it seemed the battle was lost.

Nora was used to complex environments. She had been the only westerner working at a hospital run by an oil company outside Dammam, Saudi Arabia, on 9/11. She had worked through the Iraq War there and after a brief stint back in Ireland was based in Bahrain when the hospital she worked in came under military control in the upheaval of the Arab Spring. In the Middle East, she'd dealt with SARS, uprisings, military interventions. Now she was dealing with a challenge that far surpassed all of them, far closer to home.

That January, her phone kept ringing. Contact tracers with word of another nurse taken out of action. And another. And another. The list of absentees kept getting longer while the reserves disappeared. Over an eight-week period, 'everyone was gone. You had seven, eight, maybe nine wards that were just cut out overnight.'

CUH had escaped much of the worst of the first wave. In the third wave, it would not be so fortunate. By 15 January, there were 159 Covid in-patients. Staff were redeployed from surgery theatres on to the wards, with forty doctors out of action. The exhaustion was relentless. Staff sucking air through a mask, projecting their voice through their gear to be heard by their colleagues and their patients.

Nora Twomey flipped roster after roster ripping up each draft and starting again. The goodwill of the nursing team really shone when times were bleak. 'You're switching people on days to nights, people on nights to days,' she says.

The hospital's isolation for Covid patients brought the saddest of personal stories. Husbands and wives, separated by their sickness. Other couples having to watch their beloved's funeral on iPad.

'I remember one poor woman, she was in and her husband died when she was in there. She was not well enough to go to the funeral, and couldn't go anyway because she had coronavirus,' says Professor Horgan. Another woman's husband, a few doors down from her in the same ward, died too. 'She didn't want to see him. She wanted to remember him as he was.'

The staff had to battle to maintain connections. Calling families every day to say: 'Look, Mrs Murphy, she's doing fine, we just want to let you know she's stable.' Allowances were made to get family members in if someone was dying in isolation. These were the most heartbreaking calls to make. 'We had one woman who had flown in from a city in the UK to her mother's funeral. She infected her aunt and uncle-in-law and the three of them ended up in hospital,' says Professor Horgan.

The nature of the post-Christmas Covid infection in the early days of 2021, noticed by the staff of CUH, spoke to a far wider spread of the virus than the previous waves. In March and April and in the October wave, West Cork, for example, did not see as many patients admitted to CUH as the urban areas. Staying on top of things was not easy. One morning Mary Horgan saw a patient and was puzzled. She asked staff: 'Hang on, I thought we'd discharged that woman.' It turned out to be the woman's twin sister, admitted just after her sibling had been discharged.

One man with Covid, Professor Horgan remembers, was panicking, suffering with lung failure. 'The nurse was really upset too. We had to obviously manage the patient first, to make sure he was as comfortable as possible – but to ensure the nurse was okay too.' The struggle to keep distressed patients comfortable was a traumatic experience for staff, Professor Horgan says, especially for younger staff members.

The Irish Nurses and Midwives Organisation was particularly concerned about CUH during the surge, noting the 'extreme pressure' the hospital was under, including the intensive care unit, which was full to the brim. Mary Horgan says 'there were at least three hundred nurses out' at the peak of the wave in January. 'We had at one point over forty trainee doctors out.' It was chaotic. 'Everything nearly had to close down.'

'When does it end?' she asked. With staff at a premium, resources depleted and tragic stories unfolding around them, the women and men of CUH battled against it all to keep going.

* * * *

From the back room of his family home, Tony Holohan adjusted his webcam and joined the Zoom call. It was

Christmas Day. There were some gripes among those logging on. The CMO knew it was a sore spot because they didn't mention the meeting for a few weeks to come. 'Sorry, guys, we've no choice in the matter,' Holohan told them. Things were that bad.

There were daily video meetings between Holohan and his inner circle, as well as the broader membership of NPHET. Holohan, turkey in the oven, settled in for the meeting, with special advisor to NPHET and one of the CMO's closest colleagues Darina O'Flanagan, Cillian De Gascun and Fergal Goodman among the tight-knit group on the call.

That festive season was a painful one for Holohan. He knew it would be his final Christmas with his wife, Emer, and their children as a family. There was precious little quality time for them. 'I felt terrible, personally.' Christmas was taken over, dominated by teleconferences, epidemiology meetings, NPHET conferences and multiple briefings to Government and the sub-committee. 'This is how I was spending it,' he says. 'I couldn't do anything about that. I was in it and that was it. So, yeah, my feelings about that are fairly complex, you know?'

He felt guilty about disrupting other NPHET members' Christmases too. The plan had been to strip back their meetings to allow them to have some rest before the anticipated deterioration really kicked in. It wasn't to be.

Further recommendations had been made to Government by NPHET on 23 December about what should happen from St Stephen's Day. The health system was deemed to be at serious risk of collapse and there was an obvious risk of deaths and serious illness to follow as families of younger generations came together with grandparents over Christmas. Holohan said the Government's initial moves wouldn't cut it. 'There is too great a risk in waiting to assess the measures announced yesterday,' he said in a letter to the Health Minister, urging him to implement the full suite of Level 5 restrictions from St Stephen's Day. That decision would not come from Government until 30 December.

As Tony Holohan put on his reading glasses to go through the data with his colleagues on 25 December, hundreds more families would also be having their final Christmas meals together.

Chapter 17: The Mater II

'Just please, please don't be afraid to pick up the phone and I'll be in.'

Dr Eavan Muldoon felt guilty. She felt 'extraordinarily guilty'. She phoned once, twice, three times, offering to come back to work alongside her colleagues. They were facing into the unknown in March 2020, a daily onslaught of admissions in April, and Eavan, a dedicated infectious diseases consultant, was at home on maternity leave.

She was regularly in contact with her team on the frontline. 'I felt I should have been there. I should have been in the trenches. I should have been contributing. I've a ten-year-old and now I've got an eighteen-month-old – I was clearly not expecting any more children,' she laughs. She says it was like being in a little bit of a 'bubble' for those months, worrying about her friends in the Mater, while she was taking care of her baby.

A consultant for a number of years, Muldoon had worked in the USA and the UK, returning home to Dublin in 2017. She had spent years of her career training for the possibility of a global pandemic of the magnitude of Covid-19. When it first appeared on her newsfeed, she devoured stacks of medical journals and media reports about the new 'pneumonia' outbreak in China. She was immediately interested in something that had the potential to redefine her line of work.

'You've missed it all' was a nagging thought that often crossed her mind. '*You've missed it all.*' Whenever she called the hospital to offer her services, when she got back to work in the quieter months of June, the hospital's CEO, Alan Sharp, remembers her feeling that guilt.

When she returned to her ward rounds, she was hit by a barrage of new work practices. There were different patient pathways – Covid and non-Covid; the constant conversations about getting tests back from the labs; Zoom as the main outlet for any meetings between departments. The readjustment wasn't easy. 'One of my big things is I always shake my patients' hands and introduce myself. It's kind of a social crutch maybe. All of a sudden that's gone and I'm, well, I feel really awkward. What do I do with my hands?'

Almost everyone in the Mater remembers the moment they realized Christmas and January were going to be bad. For Dr Colman O'Loughlin it was his friends' stories of standing-room only in their local pub in the suburbs of Dublin, the place hopping, car parks full, and the mandatory €9 pizzas were out the window. 'I know households and households and households that got Covid out of that pub.'

'It was a slap in the face,' says Ken A. Byrne. Ken and his mates among the porters were frustrated looking at groups of young people hanging around. 'It only takes one or two of them to have it and then what happens to someone who reacts badly to it? Where do they end up? In the hospital. Back in our laps.'

Eavan Muldoon's strange 'fomo' had long since faded. The second wave through September and October, while not overwhelming, never dropped to a 'normal' baseline. Staff in the Mater wouldn't see a quiet day from that September until the far side of April 2021. Everything from the autumn was one wave after another, breaking over them, dragging them down.

Eavan ate sandwiches in the freezing cold in her sister's back garden for Christmas Day, wary of indoor mixing. Later, as she took her baby for a walk on the streets of Drumcondra, hoping to get him to sleep for just a little while, she was shaken by the sight of car after car wedged into narrow driveways. 'There are a *lot* of people just hanging out and eating. I knew right then this would be trouble.' She was on call over Christmas and was in work for Stephen's Day and on the twenty-seventh, exchanging the usual seasonal good wishes with her colleagues. After the handover, the Mater was 'swamped' by New Year's Day. 'It exploded. It just blew up.'

Every patient admitted in to the Mater throughout the pandemic has their own story, such as Daniel, a young man under the care of Dr Muldoon, who had been working in a restaurant over Christmas. Three of his colleagues had been diagnosed but he went on working, ignoring some slight symptoms, not wanting to cause a fuss.

'I've seen 28-year-olds sitting chatting to me one day and their only risk factor might be they're maybe a little bit overweight or they've got diabetes,' she says. 'And you come in the following day and they're on four litres of oxygen and then later on that evening you're sending them up to the ICU.' The speed of deterioration over Christmas had doctors like Eavan spooked. They kept close watch, afraid that an hour away could see the people in their care fall victim.

Mary Elizabeth Jones took blood from an older woman, Margaret, who wept with guilt in her hospital bed. 'I knew I shouldn't have had them all over for Christmas dinner.' How many people was that? Fourteen. Several were now infected. 'She was blaming herself, she was so upset,' Mary Elizabeth says, the memory bringing back her own tears. 'I kept telling her, "No, people have to live. It's Christmas." Her family were on the phone non-stop and I just couldn't reassure them that she would survive. Christmas is such a celebration but all of these people suffered for it. They suffered so much.'

In the first week of January, scheduled training on St Cecilia's was quickly cancelled. This was not a drill. 'It was nothing like the first time,' says Mary Elizabeth. It was busy, patients were admitted, and more would immediately follow. In the spring, patients would only deteriorate four or five days into their time in hospital. In winter, by the time they were in the Mater, they were already in a dreadful state.

The nature of the sickness changed too. Mary Elizabeth and her colleagues were treating more patients for clotting and pulmonary embolisms. It required constant vigilance. The people who were getting sick were younger, and not all of them had the same comorbidities as the patients of the first wave. 'I couldn't explain it. I couldn't tell you who was going to get really sick and who wasn't. You'd see thirty-year-olds coming in and I'd think, "I'm thirty, how is this happening?"'

As a nursing manager, Mary Elizabeth worried about the younger members of her team. Just twenty-three or twenty-four, the nurses were thrown into hell managing a situation that they could never have prepared for. Older infectious patients became confused or delirious and wandered onto the halls in the night, thrashing out in the low light, calling out for family members or a home that seemed so distant now, causing panic for those on duty. Nurses, alone, had to manage these situations on their own. 'It's hard to rationalize what they do with people who are dying and their families,' says Clinical Director Professor Jim Egan. 'I don't know how they did it.'

Mary Elizabeth Jones would cry, sick with worry about those young healthcare workers under her. 'Are they going to be okay after all of this?' she asks, thinking of all of the nurses and students who played their part, not just in the Mater but across Ireland. She believes there'll be an exodus. 'They can all head off to Australia, the young ones, they deserve to get out after all of this. They deserve the best time of their life.'

For Ken A. Byrne and the porters, the third wave was about survival. They would stare at the entrance on the North Circular Road with steely determination and tell themselves to hold fast. 'Whatever comes through those doors, we have to deal with it'. They were exhausted and battered, but the workload grew and grew.

The best support they had was each other. One coffee break, Dr Eavan Muldoon remembers chatting with an older colleague when another consultant came into the room. 'Oh, I'm just giving Eavan some counselling,' Eavan's colleague said. 'Funny – it sounded like she was counselling you,' said the consultant, observing what was actually happening in the room. 'Isn't that what we do?' she says. 'We provide that kind of sounding board for each other.'

The nurses kept going too. Their role often made them the bearers of despair. They reasoned with families, trying to explain why their loved one could not have someone in to hold their hand or whisper gently in their ear. It brought no end of sadness.

St Cecilia's medics were adamant from the start that no patient of theirs would die alone. Nurses and doctors often took fifteen-minute shifts to watch over older patients as they quietly slipped away. Mary Elizabeth Jones lay in bed at night, awake and worried that her patients would not have someone with them in their final moments. 'I think it'll take a while to break that down in the future.'

For social worker Heather Hawthorne, one patient will always stay with her. Mildred, a woman in her nineties, was admitted to hospital. Her family were constantly in touch to try to find out how their beloved granny, who lived with them, was doing. They sent in emails of photos and cards to be printed out for her room. Heather remembers looking at the photos of Mildred and her family, nestled in cuddles, heads touching together with glowing smiles painted across their faces. 'She was so loved.

I thought she would be our miracle case.' Heather kept the family in the loop, phoning them every single day to let them know how Mildred was doing – if she was sleeping, what she was eating. There was no prospect of a visit; all the family had been infected with Covid at that stage. 'She was doing really well, day to day,' she says. 'And then all of a sudden she wasn't, unfortunately.'

When she died, it had a major impact on Heather and everyone who had come across her on their daily rounds, growing attached to her and the family in those pictures around her bed. Those still frames, tiny glimpses into the lives they led before this living nightmare descended on all of them, and took from them their precious mum and granny. The staff could have spent hours filling in the blanks of her life. But then there's the next call. There was always another call. Another patient, another family counting on them to put it all on the line for them once more.

* * * *

In the ICU, Dr Colman O'Loughlin was carefully removing his goggles, sliding gloves off his hands. Another day of unrelenting pressure was over and another would soon begin. He counted the cost as he trudged back to the car park. On the worst days, the Mater's ICU team would take two, three or four critically ill admissions. Sitting in his car, he'd give himself a moment to try to make sense of the numbers before turning the key in the ignition. 'My God,' he'd think. 'If we see the same again tomorrow, we're done for.'

The attrition was merciless. In the first wave, perhaps twenty per cent of people brought into ICU died from Covid. In the third, that figure all but doubled, surging to thirty-five per cent, says Colman. There was no breathing room, no break from the virus that was everywhere they turned. Across the

ICU, every patient was Covid. His staff members went down with Covid. His hands were washed raw to stop himself from taking it home.

'It was very wearying,' says Colman. His colleagues watched patients die; many others who survived were left with lasting physical damage – many requiring oxygen for a long time afterwards, their lungs scarred and tarred by the disease. 'We were trying to help them as best we can,' he says, 'but we're not able to help them as much as we could help with other diseases.' It was a psychological gauntlet. Their minds warped to blame themselves. 'It almost felt we weren't doing our job well enough.'

The ICU in the Mater was taking in some of the most critically ill ICU patients not just in Dublin but from across the country. Mobile ICU ambulances criss-crossed the map, transferring patients hundreds of kilometres for life-saving treatment when their nearest hospital exceeded capacity. For some, it was their final journey; for others it was a precarious journey to a treatment of last resort.

The Mater is the only hospital in the country, and one of only six between Ireland and Britain, equipped with extracorporeal membrane oxygenation or ECMO. It's an ultra-aggressive form of intensive care, beyond even ventilation. Thick, translucent pipes go into the patient's body, drawing blood out, pumping oxygen through it and back into the body. In effect, as Colman O'Loughlin explains, it creates a mechanical heart and lungs outside the body. The patient's vital organs are taken out of the equation, bypassed in the hope that it gives them a chance to heal. 'It has a very low survival rate. These are the sickest of the sick. You're talking about a forty or fifty per cent survival rate on ECMO.' Extra staff are needed to monitor ECMO beds, a tireless vigil, while family members wait in desperate hope for a recovery that may never come.

Throughout the hospital, the staff stood up. Non-consultant

doctors would stand in for their senior colleagues. 'I'm twenty-eight. I'll do this,' they'd plead. 'There's no point in you going in as a sixty-three-year-old.' They took on the task and rolled up their sleeves and fought with a responsibility far beyond their years. Colman believes many great doctors were forged in the fire of the third wave. Their consultant colleagues were awed by their courage. They gave more than anyone could ever ask of them.

It was not an easy burden. Ken A. Byrne would be on the 122 bus from Cabra every morning, hitting the stop button on the North Circular Road, ready to start work at 10.45 in the morning. He'd work through until eight o'clock, weaving through HCAs, cleaners and student nurses all moving through the gates, and get back on the same bus home.

'It was very, very hard not to take it home,' he says. He'd sit on the sofa, open a can of Heineken, turn on the news and hear about people dying, and would think back to patients he had met over the course of the day. What their name was. What their fears were. He never stopped thinking and worrying about the patients. 'Jaysus, I hope one of them isn't that lady I met earlier,' he'd fret. The feelings were heavy to carry, but at the same time, 'I'd rather go home and feel like that, because at least then I'm having the right feeling. I'm sitting there thinking about the patients and I hope to God they're alright.' It reminded him that he was only human.

One element of the last year that has stuck with Colman O'Loughlin and the ICU team is self-harm. There's no question in their mind that there has been an increase in the number of patients the department has seen with deliberate instances of injuries caused at their own hand. 'There's no doubt about that; especially in the first wave, we saw more of it,' says O'Loughlin. 'We often don't see it bad enough that it comes to intensive care. To come to intensive care, you're risking your life.'

There were patients who came through with severe drug overdoses. There were patients who came through with suicide attempts. O'Loughlin points to the fact that research shows the number of suicides hasn't increased by any large degree on previous years, but his staff do believe that, at least in Dublin's inner city, there were more cases of deliberate self-harm, possibly out of the exclusion and isolation that lockdown brought with it. It is something, he says, that warrants reflection when the pandemic has long subsided. 'I'm married with four kids, my life didn't change all that much', but for others who may have lived alone and missed the outlet of work or social clubs, the impact was far greater. Lockdown 'was absolutely for the right reasons, for the greater good of the population, but in time it may turn out to be a huge problem. The mental health services are going to have a huge job of work to do when they're back in full flow again.'

No one who worked at the Mater Hospital wasn't changed by the experience of Covid-19. It's impossible not to carry the weight of responsibility, the long hours, the tears, the trauma, the pain and struggles through PPE, the pressure marks from goggles worn for hour after hour, the personal battles won and lost over the long months that did not end.

The WHO declared 2020 'The Year of the Nurse'. To outsiders, this may have seemed a trite gesture, but it recognized the world's gratitude to those women and men who put themselves at risk, often at the expense of their own lives, to protect the vulnerable and frightened.

On 12 May 2020, the Mater's nursing staff came together, at distance, on the corridors of the Whitty Wing for a brief ceremony. There, in front of noticeboards carrying Thank You cards from the public, from patients and their families, and from the local primary schools, they came to reflect on what had been done and what was to come. A small red varnished wooden box was produced. Suzanne Dempsey stood, projecting her voice so that her socially distanced colleagues could hear how proud she was of them all. The box was a time capsule, to be opened again on 12 May 2120. Books of memories, thoughts, lived experiences were collected and put in the box. Some included pencil sketches of themselves both in and out of their PPE and visors, the tight and sometimes foggy lens through which the biggest challenge of their lives unfolded before them, hour by hour.

It's not hard to imagine the excitement the nurses of 2120 will feel when they finally get the chance to open it, laughing, smiling, eager to learn about the predecessors who shared laughter and tears together just like them, who came to work and gowned up every day, who lived through a chapter of history that will be remembered for many generations to come. The Mater's stated hope is to one day have a heritage centre within the hospital where the public can dive in to the archives and eyewitness accounts of the people who looked after Dublin's sick. Until then, those deepest thoughts and memories will go unread.

When the staff of 2120 come to hear about the battles fought by Mary Elizabeth Jones, the strength and leadership of Suzanne Dempsey, the quiet care of Patricia Prades, the compassion and smiles of Ken A. Byrne, the thoughtful dedication of Eavan Muldoon, the extra mile travelled by Heather Hawthorn, they will be learning from our best.

Management thinks back on the history of the Mater – still standing, still a heartbeat in the centre of the capital; a history that now includes this prolonged period of tragedy that asked so much of its staff. CEO Alan Sharp goes back through the milestones – the epidemics of the 1800s, the 1918 pandemic, the Easter Rising, the War of Independence and Civil War, the Dublin bombings and the Stardust fire. 'There's been many a footnote around very difficult times that the Mater has helped to care for people,' he says. 'This is going to be another exceptional moment in the history of the institution, where it did its part in caring for people not just from Dublin but around the country, where we supported and cared for our patients in the best way we possibly could.'

Chapter 18: Armageddon

Government Buildings, Dublin, January 2021

Micheál Martin's Christmas had been a short one. Between the last-minute Brexit deal on Christmas Eve and the worsening Covid crisis of skyrocketing cases and hospitalizations, the Taoiseach had to hold the fort during perhaps the most turbulent festive period any Government had encountered.

He consulted with his favoured experts late into the night. He sounded out Professor Mary Horgan, added to NPHET in December. He checked in on what UK-based experts like Dr Susan Hopkins of Public Health England, originally from Kildare, had been saying about the new variant. He scrolled through message after message in a WhatsApp group set up by clinicians that he was added to back in March. He wouldn't message the group, but dipped into the research papers the members shared. When he took to his feet on 30 December to announce a return to full Level 5 restrictions, the Taoiseach laid the blame squarely on the UK variant. 'On Christmas Eve, we received the news we had feared – confirmation that the new strain is indeed in our country,' he said. It was an extraordinary conclusion to make before any major genome sequencing had been carried out, and many in NPHET were aghast at the definitive nature of his statement when there was little data to support his claim.

The meetings with NPHET over Christmas took him back to the Sycamore Room. For Martin, it's the visual memory he says his mind will snap back to whenever he thinks about the pandemic in years to come. Far removed from the bustling tumult of the first cabinet sub-committee under Varadkar's government in March 2020, it was now all but empty. The Taoiseach sat there, with a handful of his closest colleagues and advisers. Gone was the bluster of the showdowns of October and November; the Taoiseach and Martin Fraser were left to pick up the pieces of a country in turmoil. The Sycamore Room is 'where the dredge and drudgery' was, he says. 'All the meetings, the lads were beaming in. Tony's beaming in. Paul's beaming in. Philip's beaming in. You've a load of Secretary Generals looking in.'

To Leo Varadkar, 'the horse had left the stable'. On 22 December, he had predicted 2,000 cases per day by New Year's Eve and was met with a few dubious looks from colleagues, who privately thought he was being dramatic. For Eamon Ryan, it was like 2010 all over again. A veteran of the Fianna Fáil–Green Party coalition that oversaw the financial crash and the EU-IMF bailout, Ryan had been in this room before in days of crisis, rumours and desperate scrambles. 'It was scary,' he says, as senior ministers watched the admissions to hospital tick towards their limits and the numerical brutality of exponential growth. 'It's similar to that November 2010 feeling, yeah, shit this is very scary.'

As Ireland faced into a New Year wrought with human catastrophe, another spat between NPHET and Government was festering online. Dr Cillian De Gascun, tweeting late at night on New Year's Day, said that the UK variant was appearing in fewer than ten per cent of samples that had been sequenced to date, rebutting the Taoiseach's claims. Driving the point home, he said 'it is not responsible for the recent significant & concerning increase in #SARSCoV2 case numbers.'

Internally, the Government went ballistic. Senior officials and ministers couldn't believe that they were being openly contradicted by a member of their advisory team. They believed De Gascun was playing politics and many sensed the hand of Tony Holohan. De Gascun and Holohan deny that they coordinated the tweet, which was described by a senior member of NPHET as massively inappropriate and provoking an unnecessary backlash from the politicians. It's understood that Holohan and De Gascun had discussed the prevalence, or lack thereof, of the UK variant beforehand, though Holohan denies instructing his colleague to send the tweet. Professor Mary Horgan, De Gascun's colleague on NPHET since being added to the group by the Health Minister in December, quote-tweeted him saying that it was a premature statement. The move created some level of tension between the pair, with De Gascun privately telling colleagues he had been undermined but stood by the data. Leo Varadkar, for his part, says the variant was 'not a major factor pre-Christmas.' It was still only in the foothills of its ascent here. Soon it would become a mountainous challenge, but not yet.

The row about the variant would continue, but it was a battle for another day. In the trenches of frontline healthcare, as politicians and officials whispered in anonymous briefings against each other, the real battle was just beginning.

Micheál Martin was worried. His biggest anxiety was whether the system would hold. The HSE's Paul Reid, in his communications with Government at least, tried to convey a sense of calm. The Taoiseach, reading the 'vibes' he was picking up from the HSE chief in multiple phone calls, felt the ICU capacity situation was teetering on the edge of ruination. 'Armageddon' is what the Taoiseach had deemed it in his mind. 'Can we avoid Armageddon in losing control of it within the hospitals?' It was 'touch and go'. And ministers were very alarmed at the trajectory. Leo Varadkar felt things were now 'far too close for comfort'. Ministers kept a close eye on the figures as new cases and ICU admissions ticked higher and higher towards the point of no return.

'We came so close,' says Paschal Donohoe. 'We came so close to terrible, terrible, terrible difficulties.' The images of Italy from the first wave were the source of the Government's terror. The prospect of a collapsing health system and mass death were active concerns. Would the streets of Limerick or Cork become Ireland's Bergamo? It was a very real fear and it felt like control was slipping from the authorities' hands. Even two bad days of admissions, or two more bad days of uncontrolled community transmission, could have seen the emergency rocket into an even graver space.

The January meetings of Cabinet were very solemn affairs. Ministers, in the meeting rooms or remotely, sat in glum silence as the gravity of the toll was spelled out to them. 'We had etched into all of [our minds] the fact that we made decisions that had contributed to it,' says Donohoe. 'We were all aware of that.'

For many ministers, the first wave didn't affect people they knew. They were aware of their responsibilities but they were not confronted, in many cases, with the human loss at the centre of this pandemic. That changed in January 2021. The Taoiseach was hearing about people he knew dying. His wife, Mary, would call letting him know that neighbours and friends of theirs were very sick. He'd ring them to express his condolences and listen to them talk about their loved ones' experiences. Some of the calls are understood to have been with the relatives of older people who were pining to get out and meet people. 'Some of his calls were awful' says one of the Taoiseach's advisors, 'he was hearing some very sad stories of elderly people saying "I want to be with the family on Christmas Day." That's the saddest thing. They got Covid. They passed away.' It weighed on him. He won't talk about the calls he made but, reflecting on their losses, he acknowledges he felt pain for them. 'You are down,' he says. 'You're very down about the whole thing. That sort of experience must be very difficult for families.'

Leo Varadkar, keeping in touch with colleagues in medicine, was extremely worried about ICU capacity. 'I remember one of my lines throughout the year had been: we never came close to running out of beds or running out of oxygen, or ventilators, or ICU capacity. We never came close until January. And when we did it was far too close for comfort.'

Over in NPHET, the contributions of frontline medics conveyed sheer terror to the CMO and his colleagues. The underestimation of the R number going into Christmas played on the mind of Professor Philip Nolan and his colleagues. Now they were watching the ICU figures every day with growing dread. Ireland was on the very brink of a total capitulation.

There are some who say Ireland survived the third wave without ever exceeding capacity or pushing past a point of no return. They say we didn't 'go over the cliff' – drawing comparisons with Bergamo in the spring of 2020, or India in early 2021.

To other people's minds, however, we did go over the cliff. Hospitals, particularly those beyond Dublin City, were forced to treat critical patients outside ICU; they were forced to make decisions about whether ICU care would or could be extended to some patients and not to others. To these people, including senior people on NPHET, this is the very picture of a health system overwhelmed. One of them is Dr Ronan Glynn. The Deputy CMO says that Ireland 'did go over the cliff'. He repeats: 'We *did*.' The public, despite being all too aware of the crushing consequences of the surge in their own families, communities and local hospitals, were not privy to the big picture.

The burden of responsibility was damaging to the staff at the Department of Health. Officials across all levels speak of low-level anxiety in the quieter times, replaced by thunderous emotional burnouts in the more challenging times.

For some the breaking point came at Christmas. Scrolling down through ever-lengthening pages of deaths from Covid in the HPSC figures became overwhelming. 'I had days where I couldn't stop bawling,' says one official. 'I had to take two weeks off and have a little bit of a nervous breakdown. When you're at the frontline of this, you feel a huge responsibility. Then if you have to admit defeat, you feel you're letting a lot of people down.'

Politically, the pressure was on to account for Ireland's infection rate, now the highest in the world. Later that month, at a European Council meeting, German Chancellor Angela Merkel had taken keen interest in what was happening in Ireland and quizzed Micheál Martin. Merkel, who holds a PhD in quantum chemistry, looked at our case count with a scientist's eye. 'The graph went through the roof and she saw "variant" straight away,' says the Taoiseach. Europe's leaders were shocked by what they saw in Ireland. They agreed that Ireland's Covid cycle appeared out of sync with the continent's.

'We hadn't experienced the severity that they experienced prior to Christmas,' says Martin, 'but by hell we got it after.' The Irish data alarmed both Merkel and France's Emmanuel Macron and forced them to take Europe to a new phase to ward off the havoc of the variant. Ireland's Christmas disaster was what prompted a change of heart that saw the EU finally decide that enough was enough and impose travel restrictions.

The political backlash at home was immense. Even from within the Government parties. One former minister says, 'It's something which they're going to have to live with. I think they should get the blame for that, and I hope they've learned their lesson. The Government has been playing God with people's lives and I don't think God would be too impressed with what they did at Christmas.'

Members of NPHET remember the dark January briefings when they heard reports from ICUs relayed through Dr Michael

Power, the HSE's Clinical Lead for Intensive Care, and felt helpless to intervene. There were days when NPHET members would log off the Zoom call and sit in silence staring at the blank computer screen. 'We were witness to a national tragedy,' says one member, under condition of anonymity, 'and there wasn't a thing we could do about it.'

Dr Mary Favier, sitting on NPHET and running her GP surgery, testifies to the unrelenting nature of January. 'It was never made public,' she says, 'but we had lost control of it. We now didn't have enough ventilators and there were people queuing up on corridors.' Over a four- or five-day period, and by a combination of miraculous luck and the shocked retreat of the public into lockdown and social distancing, people pulled it back. The modellers and the top table of NPHET could see the peak as Ireland passed 8,000 cases in a single day – a figure none of them had modelled or foreseen – and saw the cases slowly, slowly start to decrease. The hospital crisis did not decelerate, however.

'I felt very sorry for him,' says Favier of Dr Michael Power. 'All the intensive care specialists were losing the plot. It really looked like we weren't going to get ahead of it and the hospital service would fail.'

In hospitals across the country, the HSE's ground force converted high dependency units into temporary ICUs. High-flow oxygen was administered to the most in-need patients who could not be accommodated in ICU. At the peak, 212 people were formally in ICU. Another 320 people were on advanced respiratory supports. The HSE's CEO, Paul Reid, was 'scared', he admits. 'Moving through the second or third week of January, you just didn't think it was going to stop. I was probably more scared in that third wave than I was in the first wave.'

Some hospitals, already at full capacity in ICUs, transferred their patients to critical care units elsewhere that had space. 'There was talk of transferring people out of the country,' says

Mary Favier. NPHET members looked to Europe, where ICU patients from the Netherlands and France had been medically evacuated by military plane to hospitals in Germany. This was something they desperately wanted to avoid here.

ICU consultants in certain hospitals, says Dr Favier, 'spent all morning on the phone trying to ring all the different units to see if anybody had any bed or even any chance that somebody's died that would free up a bed. That type of stuff where you're looking for people to be dead. We got away with it, and it's not public knowledge and it didn't need to be. But it was pretty hairy.' It is a shocking admission and points to the desperation of the situation ICUs found themselves in. To free beds to keep people alive, there was almost a hope that others who wouldn't make it might die to give others that chance.

Dr Vida Hamilton, coordinating the HSE's critical care response, was watching some of the biggest units in the country fall into jeopardy, CUH and St James's in particular. To her mind, 'if either of those big units that were in trouble had fallen over – because it only takes a few people to do that – the knock-on effects on all the other ICUs' could have taken out the entire system. It was the finest of margins.

By 18 January, 2,020 people were being treated in hospital for Covid; 199 people were fighting for life in ICU, more than one hundred of them on ventilators, with machines pumping breath into their lungs. Dr Tony Holohan made a public projection that we might see 1,000 deaths confirmed in the month of January alone. Some of the commentary around deaths was eating away at him. 'Our primary duty is to stop people being killed by the virus. It's not okay to say these people were at a certain age, or had certain underlying illnesses. Their lives ended prematurely as a result of this infection. We all have private lives, and many of us are at a certain age where our parents are older. My parents are still living and they're in their early eighties, they would be statistics to many people. They're both hale and hearty and living life. Their lives won't go on for ever but their lives have value. It's amazing how that's just been discounted by people; by some people at least.

'The UK variant, even if everything else was perfect, would have presented us with an additional problem ... that would have had an impact on mortality. But we had a much, much bigger experience of mortality than we needed to have. We had over two thousand deaths between January and February in this country. I think we could have avoided a lot of that.'

Belmullet, County Mayo, January 2021

The last time Sean Conroy saw his father was at the Christmas dinner table.

Both Sean and his wife started to feel unwell the following Tuesday. When they got back from the Castlebar testing centre on New Year's Eve, an hour's drive out and an hour back, 'I was so ill, I fell in the door of the house.' That night he woke up and crawled across the hall, pulling himself to the front door, desperately gasping for oxygen, his head flat against the cold floor. 'I just lay down on the tiles and let the air come into my face to get oxygen. I was that sick.'

The Conroys are a welcoming family. Sean is the sort of man who'd go out of his way to help a stranger he'd met a minute before, the kind who'd insist that if you were ever out in Belmullet, you'd stay with them. The family ran a local pub and a local funeral directors, and had been lynchpins of the educational development of the area over the decades. Sean had to step back from the family's funeral director business while he battled Covid. A cousin stepped in to run the show. The business was overwhelmed in what was becoming a horrifying episode for the community.

Of all the deaths that visited Belmullet in early 2021, perhaps it was the passing of Bernie McAndrew that touched the community most of all. She was a local figurehead; people say she was a joy to be around and a vibrant, happy soul. She died at home, a week after she and her husband were diagnosed with Covid. The death of a young woman, a member of so many committees and a local golf club stalwart, left the Erris community irreparably heartbroken. As Bernie's body was taken from her home by hearse, her husband, Ian, now seriously ill, was transferred by ambulance to hospital. Their paths, intertwined for so many years, diverged for the last time.

'It was very traumatic on the whole town,' says Dr Fergal Ruane. 'Bernie was involved in the golf, everybody knew her. She worked in the hospital ... and she was a young woman, that really hit the town.'

Fr Michael Reilly, the parish priest, had become sick with Covid, and Fr Kevin Hegarty stepped in for funeral duties. There were many upsetting moments. 'I remember being at one funeral and seeing the ambulance pass by to bring somebody from the neighbourhood to hospital,' he says. 'People in the area were very, very upset. They couldn't attend funerals' – which were limited to ten people – 'they wanted to reach out to the bereaved. What we took as normal in the community had ended.' The wake, the sharing of stories until late at night over sandwiches and a parting glass, and the warmth of being held close by your home community when you needed it the most was ripped away and cruelly absent.

Days after the funeral of Bernie McAndrew, Sean Conroy's father, Paddy, was taken by ambulance to Castlebar Hospital. He spent a week in a stable condition, while his beloved wife of fifty-two years, Mary, was at home with a positive Covid diagnosis. The Conroy family's lives were turning upside down. All except Padraic, Sean's brother, were sick with Covid. Funeral after harrowing funeral put huge stress on them. For a short time, Sean himself was unsure whether or not he would make

263

it through his illness. Between the Monday and Friday of that week, four more people were buried. Sean was called to say his father hadn't got long left. Padraic, finishing off in the grave-yard with his cousin John, went straight to Castlebar hospital to stay with his father for the final hours of his life. He had been alone for the nine days since he was admitted.

Paddy Conroy died on 15 January. This loss was another harrowing blow to a community in the midst of its blackest hour for generations. On the day of his father's funeral, Sean was finally free from isolation and able to attend. He'll never forget the sight of the people of Belmullet turning out to pay their final tributes to a man who had left an indelible mark on Erris. The eighty-one-year-old was a truly loved figure. He would help school students coming through the vocational school or from St Brendan's, which had been set up in 1982, with applications to college or for jobs at a time when employment in the region was scarce. When governments and businesses didn't give rural Mayo a chance, Paddy Conroy did. Education, efficiency and, above all, Erris were the three Es he drove into his children. Dublin, London and places further afield had gobbled up the youth of Erris. Paddy Conroy took a stand to turn the tide of emigration.

As the hearse left the family's funeral home, it stopped outside the family pub and then slowly wound its way through the town. Hundreds of people, socially distanced, wearing face masks, stood and bowed and blessed themselves as Paddy Conroy made his last journey through his home town, where he would tell anyone he'd come across, even the guy on the paper round, that he was the first man up every morning. As the funeral procession left the church, making its way through the mean-dering country roads of the peninsula, dozens more gathered, their cars pulled up to the side of the road, standing out in the wind and rain to send Paddy Conroy off, a man who had touched all their lives.

His wife, Mary, still recovering from Covid, was unable to attend his funeral. She had said goodbye to him as he left in the ambulance to Castlebar a little over a week before, thinking he'd be home safely to her in a few days. It was not to be. A family notice in the local newspaper speaks volumes of the joy he brought the family. 'To the world you were just a part, but to us you were all the world.'

The pain continued in Belmullet throughout January. On a single day, when there was little to no traffic on the roads, twelve ambulances arrived. Twelve times in one small village. GP Dr Keith Swanick told the *Irish Independent* he admitted five patients from their homes that weekend. 'An ambulance had to travel from Manorhamilton to Belmullet, another had to come from Clifden,' he said.

Fr Kevin Hegarty is a thoughtful man, known in religious circles around Ireland for his reflections and his writings. It's a trait that's seen him fall foul of Church authorities. In 1994, he was effectively sacked from *Intercom*, the Catholic Church's magazine in Ireland, for commissioning courageous and scathing articles raising the issue of clerical sex abuse and calling for inquiries. It was this outspoken nature that saw him moved back to his old home in Belmullet to work as a curate in Kilmore-Erris; a banishment, in the words of Patsy McGarry of the *Irish Times*, to a parish 'so far west you must watch your footing to avoid falling into the Atlantic'.

For Fr Kevin, the outbreak was a lonely experience. 'I felt helpless. I just wish I could do so much more and be with people so much more.' The support of other priests was harder to come by. Isolation and funeral after funeral had an impact, but he kept doing what his vocation asked of him and made sure he comforted as many grieving families as he could. 'I have no easy answers for you,' he'd tell them. He pressed family members to avoid blaming themselves for how the virus may have been contracted but to lean on each other. 'One thing

I kept on stressing to people – I said, I'm not going to try and make any easy predictions for the future. But I do have a sense that the next few weeks are going to be difficult in the community because of the spread of the infection.'

The sight of people lining the streets and roads of Belmullet is one that will perhaps haunt the Erris community for a long time to come, but there was solace to be found in those moments as hundreds of people stood tall together to show their respect for the lives that were lost. It is no exaggeration, in Hegarty's view, to say that it was a communal suffering not seen in the area since Famine times. 'That brought tears to many eyes on those wintry, sad days, that people stood out as a coffin made its way to the graveyard.' In a way, Fr Hegarty hopes this practice will continue at funerals to come, a public demonstration of a community united in grief.

As January gave way to February, the snowdrops finally brought new life to the desolate hills, but whispering and rancour continued in an Ireland that had become, once again, the Valley of the Squinting Windows. It's something journalist Aoife Grace Moore noticed regularly, contrasting the level of 'curtain twitching' that went on in the Republic with the 'say nothing' culture in her home place of Derry, where people 'minded their own business'. Locals and businesses complain of their names being blackened after Christmas, some almost afraid to show their faces in the village for the opening months of the year.

Sean Conroy often wonders about the impact on people who, like himself, his sister and his mother, couldn't say goodbye to their loved ones who died in hospital. 'They had to go to a funeral with a closed coffin and … really even wonder is that their husband who has been laid to rest in that grave there? You know, because so many victims came out of mortuaries at the same time. There's always that psychology involved in it.' He still holds on to hope. 'Belmullet has been historically badly hit by emigration. Suffering. Loss. People have resilience. It's a generational thing and it's inbuilt.'

In quieter moments, however, he realises he himself is not over it. 'Those who are mourning their loved ones right now, they've gone through trauma that hasn't been experienced for generations here,' says Fr Hegarty. 'We don't know how that will affect them.'

O'Donovan & Son Funeral Directors, Sallynoggin, County Dublin, January 2021

Michael O'Donovan didn't sleep. The phone would ring at all hours. He couldn't believe it. Another family bereaved. Their muffled cries crackling over the phone speaker.

The first Covid funeral in O'Donovan & Sons was at the very beginning of the pandemic. Several more followed through April, but nothing on the scale of what was to come in January 2021.

Over Christmas and New Year, Annabeg Nursing Home in Ballybrack had been hit by a major outbreak, with multiple cases and deaths. Loughlinstown Hospital, too, struggled to cope. So did Carysfort Nursing Home on Arkendale Road.

Over a two-week period in January, Michael O'Donovan carried out a total of thirty-nine funerals. Twenty-four of them were Covid-19-related. It was the most strenuous, most stressful and most harrowing time in the many years he has worked in the funeral business.

He would start work every morning at half past six, donning his black tie and suit without fail. His eyes were baggy and bleary from lack of sleep. Over the coming hours, his phone would be attached to his ear. He handled calls from distressed families, from his staff as they navigated the intricacies of body removal from hospitals and nursing homes, and from the hospitals themselves, as he tried to make sure that his staff were safe and that if there was any chance a funeral could be done in person with an open coffin, that it would happen.

He'd drive home some time after 11 p.m. Or later. His brief hours of sleep would be interrupted by the buzz of his phone. Family after family. 'All through the night,' says his partner, Nicole, who works alongside him at the funeral directors' modern office in Sallynoggin village. 'For just one family's funeral, you could have twenty or twenty-five phone calls.'

Conversations with families who have lost someone they loved deeply are never easy, but in January 2021 it was harder than ever. The silence at the end of the phone told its own story. 'That's when they don't want to tell you what they're meant to tell you,' says Michael. 'They know that once they tell you it's Covid, and they've been with their loved one, they can't see the body any more after that.' Close contacts were ruled out of funerals. Many families didn't want to tell the undertaker they had been around their loved one in the days before they died, often lying about whether they'd seen their relative. They were bereft and inconsolable and wanted, quite naturally, to go to the funeral.

But rules were rules. Michael and Nicole had staff to protect. They checked in with nursing homes and hospitals asking the awkward questions to see if visitors had been admitted to see people whose funerals they were chosen to handle.

It was painful. One son, George, kept vigil by his mother's bedside before she died. He did what any son would want to do, and what his mother would want him to do, in her final hours. A crushing conversation had to be had. He would not be allowed into the funeral home; he wasn't permitted to set foot inside the church. Instead, George stood outside the church walls, listening to his mother's funeral over the speakers, watching along on his phone screen. A little more than three weeks later, George stopped by the funeral home to pay the bill. 'Ah, George, come in,' Michael welcomed him. It was in the middle of this interaction, this burdensome moment all families must go through, that it hit George. 'It's mad.' He shook his head. 'You wouldn't let me in to see off my own mother, but you'll let me in to pay the bill.' It's a moment that Michael wishes wasn't so. 'How right was he?' he asks.

Some families opted to skip the funeral service altogether, upset by the cold arithmetic of picking which relatives would make the cut. In those situations, Michael and his staff would often be asked to drive the deceased's remains in a hearse past the family home. There, the bereaved and their neighbours could come together as the hearse came to a stop.

At one such funeral in Sallynoggin, the deceased's daughter turned down a church service for her mother. 'What's the point if there are only ten people allowed in?' The family decided instead to plan a service at a later date. The croaking pain in their hoarse voices will stay with Michael. So too will the day they drove the hearse past the house. 'I'll never forget the daughters grabbing the sides of the hearse. Never ever. And screaming to try to get in to their mother.'

'There were just so many bodies,' Nicole says. It was not a straightforward process either. Sometimes bodies were released by hospitals that were only later confirmed as having had Covid. The stress of the situation was too much for some of Michael's staff, who became fearful for the safety of vulnerable family members at home.

The better nursing homes they worked with would supply PPE for the funeral directors, allowing them to swap their masks and gloves before entering. When remains were to be removed, they were already in body bags. The duty then fell to Michael's staff to put a second body bag on the remains before closing the coffin. 'We wouldn't see the body at all for Covid deaths. We have to seal the coffin there in front of them [the hospital or nursing home staff] to make sure that, when we leave, they can categorically state to the HSE that the coffin was sealed.'

Often late notification of Covid after a body has been released mistakenly in the clear has caused distress for families and O'Donovan's team alike. One young man with a severe underlying health condition died in hospital, and his family were told there was no issue – he was free from Covid. The family relayed this to Michael but he had his suspicions. The hospital was soon in contact; they apologized and confirmed that the young man had been Covid positive. Michael recoiled when he heard. It was now his role to relay that news, ripping up a family's plans to send off their son. 'It took them hours to get their heads around it. It was terrible,' he says.

There were times that gave Michael strength too. Moments he could call upon for resilience when it became too much to bear. Without them, he could simply have given up. At one funeral, where the deceased's mother was unable to attend, the priest turned to Michael as the service concluded. The plan had been to send the procession past the mother's home, where she was cocooning with an underlying condition. 'Give me five minutes. I want to go ahead of you.' The priest had had a brainwave. 'When we got there,' Michael says, 'there must have been a hundred people lined up and down the road.' The priest was there in the middle of the street waiting for them. He did a fifteen-minute service in front of the home, the neighbours, heads bowed, remembering a son of the community lost to an enemy none saw and all struggled to understand. 'It was done for the mother. It was genuinely lovely,' Michael says, 'one of the most heart-warming moments over a bad year.'

Tallaght Hospital, February 2021

'When somebody dies, I write a letter.'

Dr Anthony O'Connor had retreated to his office seeking a few moments of peace. Burying his face in his hands, he sat at his desk and remembered the patients he had lost. Thinking back for a personal memory of each of them. Thinking of some words of comfort to share with their families. Thinking of some thanks to give them for placing the care of their relative with him. 'I might normally have to do five or six [letters] a year,' says O'Connor, a consultant gastroenterologist who had been moved to Covid care early in the pandemic. 'In February I did nine.'

Some of those he treated for Covid had chronic illnesses, people he'd treated regularly for years. Many of them died over the course of the year. One woman, a patient he had a 'fierce affection for', he'd treated as a registrar and a consultant. 'She was kind of the bane of my life for about ten years,' he says, giving a small rueful laugh. 'She could be a very difficult person. She's gone now.' She died in January. Anthony was called in to do CPR on her on the day she went into cardiac arrest. She had been part of his life. 'I definitely saw more of her than I did of my parents over the last four or five years and she's dead now.' He stops to wonder about the void left by the passing of those who die. 'They leave a little hole for you as somebody who is peripherally involved in their life,' he says. 'You kind of wonder what holes they've left at home with their families.'

O'Connor would sit and think about these things. trying to pull those emotions and thoughts together. Every so often there'd be a bang on the door – he was needed. Someone was sick. Another staff member had been ruled out of action. 'It was very easy to feel overwhelmed,' he says. 'We had dark days at the start of 2021, you're sitting in your office trying to remember someone's favourite soccer team or their favourite book or music they might have mentioned or had with them. You know, just to put a personal touch to a letter you're writing to a grieving family.'

He hopes the families got some comfort from the letters. From his own perspective, writing them could be cathartic. A moment of reflection on the work that he and his colleagues were doing, the lives of the people he looked after through PPE. He looked back at the letters he'd written, then looked at his patient lists and worried. Who would be next? 'You kind of go: "How many more times am I going to have to do this before people wake up to how serious it is?"'

There were many times he came close to breaking point over the previous nine months. There were the conversations he had with his family and colleagues at the start of the pandemic about the risks involved. He took every precaution he could. He'd arrive home and immediately get out of his scrubs, dumping them in a bag and heading straight for the shower. He had one pair of scrubs to get into from work, and another for wearing while in work.

'I was very worried I was going to die,' he admits. His wife, Deirdre, who also works in healthcare, revised their wills at the start of the pandemic. It was a sobering moment. They had just moved house with their kids and were forced by the pandemic to get their affairs in order, just in case. Deep in Anthony's mind was that fear of death. 'I'm overweight. I'm asthmatic. I'm male,' he says. 'They were three risk factors of getting much sicker and dying, or so we thought at the start.' He kept a video diary of his experiences, just in case he ever felt he wanted to write a memoir in the future, or for his kids someday. One day, he sat in his car outside Tallaght Hospital, his hands resting on the steering wheel, staring down the lens of the camera and telling himself over and over again, 'I don't want to die … I don't want to die.'

The emotional turmoil of the pandemic was brought home when close friends and colleagues of his fell ill with the virus and became seriously unwell. As January's losses mounted, and the letters stacked up in his out tray, he felt anger. 'I've a lot of time for Micheál Martin,' says Anthony, a member of the Labour Party, 'I think he's a decent man, but his first speech in January' – in which he blamed the UK variant – 'could have been better. He went on and said "I was proven right", effectively. It would have been nice to see a bit of humility, and that came, because what I felt in December was, we'd been fucked under a bus here. We've gone through this period and seen our colleagues get sick and in intensive care, but like we're going to take this massive gamble against the best advice in the knowledge that if it all goes to shit, we'll just have to carry this on our shoulders. I was extremely frustrated. I can understand a bit more now where the politicians were coming from but I remember at the time being incredibly angered by it.'

He's not the only one. Several senior medics, nurses and doctors in the course of the interviews for this book still harbour anger towards the Government over the handling of the third wave and for the perceived lack of contrition in the aftermath.

The January surge had been fierce in Tallaght. One Saturday night on call, O'Connor saw fifteen Covid pneumonias admitted. Fifteen. He lost two patients that morning. More than nine months into the pandemic, only now was it truly revealing what it was capable of. 'We're at the gates of hell,' Anthony thought. 'We're at this all year and it's not going away. This is what hell looks like.'

Intensive care was teeming and capacity was soon breached. Vascular surgeon Professor Seán Tierney shared a photograph on Twitter of his empty theatre, reconfigured as a makeshift ICU. By 10 p.m. on the night of 9 January, mere hours after Tierney tweeted that photo, there were four patients ventilated there.

While some will remember the pandemic for the bedlam it wrought on their own lives at the outset, when everything flipped upside down, O'Connor and his colleagues say we must never forget January. 'People say "the health service survived; it kept its head above water". What does collapse look like? To me collapse looks like when you can't operate on somebody with cancer. That happened. Collapse looks like when you have multiple patients ventilated in your operating theatre. That happened. We collapsed.'

At the start of December, there had been 2,069 confirmed deaths from Covid in the Republic. By the end of January, there had been 3,307. By the end of February, there had been 4,319.

The virus's devastating impact touched homes and communities across the country, pushing health workers to their limits and beyond. But the impact was not limited to our hospitals. Even as the New Year brought the promise of respite in the shape of vaccinations, Ireland's nursing homes were forced to brace themselves once more.

Chapter 19: The Dark Night of the Soul

Dr Judith Butler stood in her kitchen, threw her hands into the air and let out a 'Yesss!' of pure relief. She had been told that her mother's nursing home was going to be one of the first in the country to welcome the rollout of Covid-19 vaccines.

It had been a year of anguished waiting, made worse by what was unfolding across the country that January. It was a year of window visits, of waving through the glass, of frantic phone calls to staff to make sure everything was okay. It had been a year of separation and of heartache. But finally, finally, it might soon be over.

Judith's mother, Noreen, was a resident in a North Cork nursing home that had escaped the first wave in April of 2020. The Christmas gift of a lifetime was the news that vaccines were coming soon. Judith excitedly texted her sister, Veronica, and brother, PJ, daily with the countdown – '5 more days to go!' Every page torn off the calendar was another day closer to safety.

Noreen was administered her first dose on 11 January. That same day, another resident tested positive for the virus. Veronica got the text confirming the news. 'Holy Mother ...', she thought. The family were instantly worried. Her mother tested positive four days later. The sharp turn from sweet relief to consuming fear was blindsiding. Visitor restrictions, as they had done for a year, prevented them from seeing their mother in her sickness. Noreen held her own for the first few days, before very suddenly becoming ill.

Every time a text alert came through, every time the phone rang, there was panic. Even when the phone didn't ring – 'Shouldn't we have heard something by now?'

Judith shared her worries with close friends. One, a nurse, suspected that Noreen might be on end-of-life care. Veronica, flustered by the news, called the home to be sure. 'Yes,' they confirmed, 'it is end of life.' They were told their mother had about two days to live.

It is a phone conversation that so many had in January, the initial heart-stopping moment leaving the family member on the end of the line in a state of shock. But there was no time to process. It was all happening so quickly. 'Our hearts were ripped from our chests and we had no control. We had just no power to help her or to do anything.'

Judith and Veronica were told not to call the home; the staff would call them. The grief was almost immediate. A local priest was organized to give Noreen the last rites over the phone. Even the rituals of life and death were conducted at a distance. The home, battling with a severe outbreak among residents and staff, asked the family to stay away. Veronica and her family said goodbye to Noreen through tears over the telephone. For Judith, this was something she simply could not do. 'I couldn't bring myself to do this,' she says. 'To this day, the thought of saying goodbye to my beautiful mother in that way upsets me so much. My heart. I couldn't do it because I was just crying so much and I didn't want my mother to have a phone held to her ear in her dying moments just to hear me crying.'

This was not the January or the New Year they had planned just weeks earlier. The final call came on the night of 23 January, just before midnight. 'My mother passed away,' says Judith, 'possibly alone, and certainly without us.'

Noreen had always told Judith that when she was dying she

must brush her hair for her and let her drift off to sleep. She always said it. 'You have to brush my hair for me, Judith.' Judith says, 'I had told her I would for the last, God, donkey's years. It was just one of those things that was ripped from us.' For Judith and so many other families, Covid took away any chance of giving their loved one the farewell they would have wanted. 'We couldn't even put on her nice clothes for her funeral, or lay her out in the coffin. She went as she was.'

In the weeks that followed, Veronica was asked to call in to retrieve her mother's belongings. 'Her life in five boxes, with a teddy bear on top,' says Judith.

Nursing homes, which navigated the first wave without sickness or deaths, found themselves overrun in early 2021. Staff and families alike have begged for answers as to why lessons were not learned from March and April.

HIQA reports into Cahercalla Community Hospice and Nursing Home in County Clare outlined a 'chaotic and disorganized' response to the outbreak there in late January. Staff were witnessed speaking to residents in a 'disrespectful and abrupt manner, speaking over residents'. One older person was observed alone 'in an isolation unit on their own five days after their requirement for isolation had passed', with little evidence of carers checking on them. Whistleblowers speaking to *RTÉ Investigates* recounted how they were told to ignore the bell if a particular resident called for help; other older people with Covid were not separated from residents who tested negative; and an outbreak of scabies was reported after staff noticed skin sores on older residents who pleaded with carers to scratch them.

HIQA inspections often happened at the worst moments. At one nursing home in the Mid-West, a GP who came in to try to help staff battling a crippling outbreak frustratedly barked at an inspector, in front of staff, to drop the clipboard and fucking help.

277

In Lusk Community Nursing Unit in north County Dublin, thirteen people died in January. The virus struck a single week before the vaccines were scheduled to arrive. The speed with which it ripped through the residents shocked Caroline Gourley, Director of Nursing with the HSE's units in north Dublin. People became seriously ill and died within days. 'If you came in contact with anything or anybody it took two and a half days and that literally was it. Every two and a half days there was another bout and there was another ... It was ... I've never seen anything like it.'

In total, 973 lives were lost in nursing homes or care facilities during the third wave of the pandemic. For Dr Ronan Glynn, it's a toll that he has yet to process. 'One of the things that has made it really difficult was that so many people died who would have been protected a few weeks later. The hardest part was knowing that these people had come through the first wave and were so close, so close to being protected.'

* * * *

The recriminations over the third wave started as Ireland came out the far side. Initially, the Government publicly stuck rigidly to the position that the UK variant was the prime factor.

Minister Stephen Donnelly, in an interview with the author for Virgin Media News, said the Government 'didn't go against public health' advice and there was 'no way of knowing' whether things would have been different if hospitality had been shut and only one visiting household had been permitted. That stance is described as 'absolute bollocks' by a senior health adviser. The view that it was all about the variant is one the Health Minister has stuck to rigidly. While NPHET did appear to underplay the role of the variant in the early days of January, until the data showed it growing in prevalence and becoming dominant, the Health Minister's assertion that it was the only reason and that socializing had no role 'is absolutely not factually correct', in the view of one senior member of the Cabinet sub-committee.

The Taoiseach appeared to be turning too. Micheál Martin admitted in February that if the Government had known then what it knew now, it wouldn't have made the same decisions. The spectre of January haunted the coalition in every restrictions decision that was to follow. Martin admits that his Government must take responsibility for its actions but becomes agitated, shifting in his chair, to make the point that he still doesn't believe that following NPHET's advice would have been the difference in preventing a third wave. 'It's a ridiculous argument, it's too simplistic. Are we seriously suggesting that first of all the broad advice is to go to Level 3? I don't buy the argument that the variations between NPHET and ourselves was the cause of it, I just don't buy that.'

His Tánaiste, Leo Varadkar, accepts some of the blame but says NPHET and the wider public weren't faultless either. He points to a combination of factors – the rise in socializing, plus foreign travel, plus the variant. A perfect storm. When he allows himself to think back over the pandemic, he believes the move from Level 5 to Level 3 was the single biggest mistake the Government made. I ask him for his view on Professor Philip Nolan's feeling, following the 26 November meeting, of guilt and despair – that they had failed to convince the Government and it was NPHET's fault. Varadkar appears surprised to hear it, blinking quickly. 'It's sobering,' he says, looking away for a moment silently.

Others feel the same: 'Rather than think it was those eejit politicians, they actually felt they had failed to convince us.' Minister Simon Harris, seen as NPHET's loudest supporter at Cabinet, summarizes his thoughts neatly: 'We have done so well in this pandemic when we've listened to the experts. We haven't done well when we haven't listened. I don't think anybody got

Christmas fully right. I think Government would concede and NPHET would concede there are lessons to be learned – like the late detection of the Alpha variant.'

While members of the 'army council' of the sub-committee do believe the Government got Christmas wrong, a responsibility they openly share, others, privately, do not believe they had any role to play in the third wave, the deaths of more than two thousand people, the hospitalization of many more and a country in a subsequent lockdown that continued for many months. These ministers ponder *who's to say* it wouldn't have been worse if the NPHET guidelines had been followed?

Putting these thoughts to members of the HSE, NPHET and the health service is an interesting experience. You're instantly met with incredulity and various inflections and emphases on the word '*Really*?'

'It's worrying. It's very worrying to hear,' says one senior HSE figure. 'They're wrong. And that's it, you know? Milton Friedman said one person with a correct argument trumps the majority opinion and they were wrong. Yeah, it was preventable.'

One key member of NPHET remains despondent. 'The biggest regret I have is Christmas,' he says. 'I don't mind the Government disagreeing but to not take ownership of it afterwards was very frustrating because Christmas was preventable. From the point of view of leadership, I found it very disappointing that they would just stand up and argue that black is white and say they took the public health advice when they obviously didn't.'

* * * *

Ireland entered the dark night of the soul. Locked down in restrictions, with the threat of Alpha still large, the country entered a period of prolonged misery that tested the patience of even the most ardent public health advocate.

Parliamentary party meetings were initially full of penance. 'One TD was screaming before Christmas saying "we have to open all the pubs,"' says one senior Fianna Fáil member, 'then in January, at one of our meetings, says "Taoiseach, you should never again listen to us, I was one of the people calling for this, please, I'm not going to say nothing again."' Within two months, the TD was once again baying for exemptions and changes to the lockdown policy.

Micheál Martin found critics even closer to home than that. He regularly faced interrogations from his kids about not sticking closer to NPHET's advice. 'What is the old man doing?' was a regular complaint, he says. His daughter Aoibhe is a 'zealot for public health', while his eldest, Micheál Aodh, pestered his father to have a crack at tightening travel restrictions and implementing Zero Covid. Martin, ruffling through worksheets as he shuttled up and down to Dublin in the back seat of the ministerial hybrid Lexus, would hear his phone bleep. Invariably, it would be another article from home. 'Have a read of this.' As the dreary months wore on, even Micheál Aodh started to ask for sport to open up. The Taoiseach gave as good as he got. 'I slag him back. I'd say "You're a hard man, I thought you were a Zero-Covider."'

Fianna Fáil also had to deal with barrages of criticism aimed at Health Minister Stephen Donnelly. Donnelly is regarded as a lone wolf, not given to trusting others in politics and 'deeply suspicious of motives', according to one person who has worked alongside him in recent years. There had been times in his early months in the job when the Taoiseach himself was frustrated by Donnelly's department. Martin fussed over delays in regulations, pushing his closest advisers to get their act together and get the Minister some help. He was delighted when the heavyweight figure of Robert Watt was finally parachuted in as interim Secretary General.

While Merrion Street was pleased the hole was plugged,

the inhabitants of Watt's new digs in Miesian Plaza fretted. He was arriving in a department of officials he had chivvied many times over the years to get spending in order. From the early 2010s, civil servants had shared stories of his notorious shouting matches in DPER with Minister Brendan Howlin, his roars reverberating through the corridors.

Once he arrived in Health, he made himself known. Occasionally, he would silently slip into the back of press conferences hosted by Tony Holohan, catching his eye, always keeping a close eye on how things were run.

Watt saw Health as a worthy challenge for an administrator of his calibre. The department once scornfully tagged 'Angola' by Brian Cowen, because of the political landmines scattered along its halls, would be a true test of his abilities. It's unlikely he foresaw some of the bizarre matters laid at his desk.

In January, Minister Donnelly queried why the Department of Health's Twitter account did not mention him. Emails obtained by the *Irish Times* and published in April showed that on a day when four thousand new cases were confirmed and Ireland was in the grip of the worst of the third wave, Watt was sent an analysis compiled by Donnelly's spokesperson Páraic Gallagher. The dossier compared Donnelly's mentions by the Department's account with other departments, such as Further Education, which regularly featured his rival Simon Harris.

While Donnelly defended the exercise, believing it to be a matter worthy of investigation, the lack of trust between the Minister and his health service was now in the open.

His scrapes with his officials were becoming legendary. At meetings with the HSE after first joining the Department, Donnelly is said by a number of people present to have misread the room badly. 'He'd come in and question things like financial management, asking "Are you sure you did that right?" He had no concept of what we'd been through as a health service throughout the first wave.'

Observers watched gobsmacked as Paul Reid, the HSE's CEO, rebuked the Minister up in front of the team. 'Reid took him to task, he said, "Oh, you know, this team has done heroic stuff in finances both before and during the pandemic and turned the place around."' It's the sort of confrontation that didn't endear him to his frontline or to the 'bureaucrats' he had lambasted for years in the national press as opposition health spokesperson. 'He didn't judge what people had personally committed to the pandemic so far and then came in and undermined them. It was bizarre to see him have to be challenged by the CEO.'

In time, Robert Watt, too, became known to admonish Donnelly in front of others. Donnelly was warned at various junctures about his public commentary and his private sugges-tions for changes in hospitals or requests to throw up new vaccination centres. 'No, no, no. That's not possible. You can't do that, Minister,' a frustrated Watt would tell him, perhaps now understanding the scale of the task on his hands.

'Donnelly doesn't have the insight or the knowledge of the public service or the civil service. He's personable and he listens, but his ability to absorb complex ideas just isn't there, in my view,' says one Health figure. 'It's certainly not right. We wanted him to do okay because we needed a good minister.'

At Cabinet sub-committee level, the Taoiseach was seen to be taking a more hands-on role in the Health agenda. Multiple sources reference one meeting where NPHET dialled in on Zoom to a sub-committee meeting in the Sycamore Room. Micheál Martin took the lead, with other senior ministers chiming in with their questions or comments. Michael McGrath, Paschal Donohoe, Eamon Ryan, Leo Varadkar ... and at the back of the line was Stephen Donnelly. 'You wouldn't have noticed he was in the meeting until that point,' says one observer. Donnelly asked vaguely about how third-level institutions would be impacted by continuing restrictions. The Taoiseach, tired and in no mood for time-wasting, was frustrated. 'You could see him tensing up,' says one witness. '"Why are you asking him that for?" he asked. The mood from Micheál was "What relevance is that?"' Another observer says, 'The Taoiseach fucking dismissed him.'

Over in Miesian Plaza, down the camera, Tony Holohan, Philip Nolan, Ronan Glynn and others could only sit and watch. The NPHET delegation was on mute. They were wearing their masks in line with public health guidance. One whispered, 'I'm tempted to say something. Talk me out of it.' Professor Philip Nolan urged quietly: 'Don't say it. Don't say it.'

Officials monitoring the meeting back at Government Buildings rolled their eyes. This was not the only time this had happened, they said. 'He's consistently performed at that level in the forum. He's always last to ask questions. And they have little relevance. He's bypassed completely.' One government official says, 'He had plenty of access to NPHET and he didn't, as far as we know, make himself available to them to kind of ask, "What are you guys going to say at the Cabinet committee?"'

It was an embarrassing moment for the Health Minister in front of his Cabinet colleagues, civil servants and the advisers back at his own department. He is described by many as 'likeable' and quick to thank people for work they do. However, he found himself increasingly bypassed, with officials in the Department of the Taoiseach pushing him, in the words of one senior official, 'to the periphery'.

'You're in the middle of a pandemic and the last person to speak in the room is the Minister for Health.' Dr Holohan and Paul Reid increasingly communicated directly with the Department of the Taoiseach, either with Micheál Martin himself, or with Martin Fraser or Liz Canavan. It's a situation that worried officials in Donnelly's own department. 'It's a risk for us. When you have a weak minister as we do with little influence, it makes our jobs fucking impossible,' says one senior staff member. 'Getting things through has just become ever more elaborate and I think it's got a lot to do with the kind of perception of weakness that there is there.'

Another says of Donnelly, 'Harris could be difficult, but basically there is no substitute for experience and Stephen Donnelly thinks he's an awful lot cleverer than he is. He doesn't understand how to use the support of his own department to get things done. He just doesn't get it. The remarkable thing about Donnelly is, you can bring him something that's good news with a bow wrapped around it and say, "Why don't you go and announce this?" And he'll either screw up the announcement or argue with you about, "Is it the right thing to do?" or be suspicious of why you're giving [it to] him, you know, "Is it ticking?"'

Members of NPHET, for their part, suspect that Donnelly does not have a strong relationship with his Chief Medical Officer. 'Tony does not suffer fools. I would say that the relationship between all of us and Stephen Donnelly is, we would love it to be professional but that would require him acting like an actual professional. He just drives us nuts. It's the bottom line. The relationship is minimal and it mostly focuses on trying to get the job done without the handicap that is Stephen Donnelly.'

Some in politics have sympathy for Stephen Donnelly. One senior member of the party says that any Health Minister under Micheál Martin has an extraordinarily difficult job. 'I have said for years and years that I'm sorry for anyone who would have been Spokesperson for Health, or Enterprise, or Education because Micheál would always jump in and say "When I was Minister, I did this." He's so quick to remind you that he was Minister and it must be quite undermining.'

One senior member of the health service says it's 'easy to pass judgement' on Donnelly, 'but a lot of people don't like him. He gets hooked on ideas that are so far off the point. His ability to focus on things of little relevance in the middle of a crisis is astonishing. I saw him once on the *Claire Byrne Show*, and all I was reminded of was Ron Burgundy in *Anchorman*.' Why? The official recalls the scene in the Will Ferrell comedy where it's discovered that news anchor Burgundy will read anything on the teleprompter. 'Then the next night they write "go fuck yourself San Diego" and Burgundy [reads it out, and then] says "that's a wrap, good show, thank you everybody." That reminds me of Donnelly, that it could be an absolute car crash and he'd be "well done everybody, that's a wrap". When he's answering questions on national television saying "I'll get back to you on that" or "Just before the show I looked this up", he just doesn't see how bad that is.'

Another official, continuing the pop culture references, says he reminds them more of Ricky Gervais' character from *The Office*. 'He comes into meetings and says things like "You know, I couldn't sleep last night guys because I was going on *Claire Byrne* this morning, so I got up at three-thirty a.m. to do a jog, about 10km, and these thoughts came to me" and he goes on. It's [got] something of *The Office*, of David Brent about it.'

Hammered, both privately and publicly, in the press and in the party, Donnelly's reputation would sink or swim on the rollout of Ireland's vaccines.

Chapter 20: The Game Changer

The Helix, Dublin City University, March 2021

The first question to be asked was whether it was possible. And the answer wasn't positive.

Dr Maitiu Ó Faoláin was tearing his hair out. The hopes of a smooth rollout of AstraZeneca vaccines to GPs was already binned by a NIAC recommendation against giving it to the over-70s. Pfizer, and to a lesser extent Moderna, were the only options now. How do you go about getting a temperature-sensitive vaccine, which had to be kept at -70°C, to 1,500 doctors' surgeries across the country? The answer is you can't. 'It was a real sense of "we're fucked,"' says Ó Faoláin.

If GPs were going to play a role in the vaccine rollout, many of them would have to figure out how to band together in large groups to limit the logistical nightmare.

Ó Faoláin's phone rang on a Sunday afternoon. He was sitting at home after a walk, looking down towards the sea. Susan Clyne from the Irish Medical Organisation was on the line. It was time to make the vaccines work. 'If you were to bring GPs together in Dublin, could you give me three buildings where that might work?' she asked. He racked his brain for suggestions. His first idea was the Covid hub in Dublin City University. He raced out there with a measuring tape trying to figure out how moving people in and out safely would work in such a confined space. A chance meeting with one of the security guards on campus held the key. 'What about the Helix?' the guard asked, pointing up towards the theatre on the Northside campus. The HSE had already acquired it as one of forty mass vaccination centres across the country, to be used later in the programme.

Ó Faoláin pounced. However, at a time when vaccines were rare and precious vials of gold dust, he came across an unlikely hurdle: 'Our patients won't go across the Liffey,' moaned one Southside doctor.

'Seriously, one GP in the Dublin 4 area pulled out of the scheme because some of his patients left his practice because they refused to cross the Liffey.' It came up repeatedly in the early online meetings. 'They were saying "my patients won't go Northside", and I said, well, they've all been to the airport and to IKEA. So we sold it to them that the Helix was right next to IKEA and the airport and everyone in Dublin had been to those two places.'

The parochial matter settled, the pace of preparations picked up considerably. By the Wednesday, Maitiu had the document drafted for the HSE. By Thursday, the HSE had given its approval. The next thing he heard was 'Can you make this happen next week?'

Scores of practices had signed up to take part that opening Saturday. Getting them all together on site in DCU was like herding cats. 'A hundred and nineteen GPs who are used to being the kings in their own ponds, all suddenly came under a system and it was so stressful.'

Finishing touches were still being made to the centre. Signs were still being thrown up to help vaccine recipients find where to check in or where to sit for observation. It was a cacophony of noisy chatter and volunteers rushing about nervously. With nine hundred people due to be vaccinated on the first morning alone, 'I had no idea if this would work, even on that first day.'

Nothing in the vaccine programme would come easily.

* * * *

Annie Lynch, from the Liberties, was the first person in the Republic to be vaccinated. She received her dose on 29 December 2020. Her family – three children, six grandchildren and two great grandchildren – were overjoyed. Her daughter Paula told the media that she was in the SuperValu car park in the lashing rain when she heard that Annie would be vaccinated. She got out of her car and ran around in the rain in joy – 'at last some good news'. Annie herself was most looking forward to a turkey dinner and a pint of Carlsberg.

The first vaccinations were the slightest break in the clouds of the third wave, but they were a break the public latched on to. We all needed hope. There were many times the hope would fade in the coming weeks and months, as Ireland stared at empty warehouses and suffered multiple mishaps.

The High-Level Task Force on COVID-19 Vaccination was commissioned in November 2020 to oversee the rollout and to coordinate the roles of the Department of Health and the HSE. Professor Brian MacCraith, a familiar face on many a public task force and commission, was picked to chair the group, which brought together the CEO of the HSE, the CMO, and officials from both the Department and the HSE. A hodgepodge of experts were mixed together to contribute, including Lorraine Nolan of the Health Products Regulatory Authority, who would be Ireland's link with the European Medicines Agency, Dalton Philips of the Dublin Airport Authority, cold chain logistics expert Derek McCormack and the IDA's Martin Shanahan. This unwieldy list of names and responsibilities had lives in their hands.

The survival of the Government was dependent on the vaccine programme. Everyone was aware of that, from Merrion Street to the HSE to the ordinary man or woman on the street. 'All you'd to do was pick up a newspaper, listen to the radio or watch the news,' says Brian MacCraith. 'It was very clear that the future of this coalition was very dependent on getting this right.' It was top billing at meetings of the parliamentary parties, which played out live on social media, such was the volume of leaking by TDs looking to get their names in the headlines. The Taoiseach and Health Minister in Fianna Fáil, and the Tánaiste in Fine Gael, would attempt to calm deputies whose backs were up about the early slow pace of the rollout. 'AstraZeneca will be coming soon and it's going to be the "game changer",' they were told. Nodding along, to convince themselves that this wouldn't be their downfall, they accepted the reassurances. 'The game changer will save us.'

Politically, there were the usual calls, ever popular in the media, for a new minister to handle the vaccination crisis. Junior Minister Ossian Smyth put his hand up for the gig. 'Eamon Ryan was actually in favour of that,' says Leo Varadkar. 'It was around the time people were calling for a minister, you know, you should have a minister for this, you should have a minister for that. Eamon put his hand up for him, he said he was willing. I never thought that was a good idea ... ultimately the HSE and the Department answer to their minister, they're not going to answer to this minister for vaccinations. That just isn't going to work.' The responsibility was left with the Minister for Health, who was managing Covid and non-Covid care, the early steps of mandatory hotel quarantine, the health regulations and, before too long, the digital Covid certificates.

Missed deliveries saw modelling shredded and started again many times. AstraZeneca, the worst offender, was the subject of a bitter geopolitical row straight from the off. On Friday,

29 January the EU moved to press the button on Article 16 of the Northern Ireland Protocol to stop vaccines moving freely into Northern Ireland from the EU. The handling of that row by Ursula von der Leyen provoked a severe backlash from politicians on both sides of the border and left many in the Government questioning whether the vaccine rollout was in safe hands. AstraZeneca missed countless deliveries to Europe, regularly underdelivering on its contracted volumes. One hundred million doses were due to be sent to the EU in the first quarter of 2021. In the end, it was only thirty million.

At the Irish end, desperation was creeping in. Paul Reid's phone, hopping under normal circumstances, erupted. He would get messages to say Ireland was expecting 52,000 doses of AstraZeneca to arrive on a given weekend. The day before the shipment arrived, a late message would come through from AstraZeneca to say it would actually be half that at 26,000 doses. The following day, as HSE procurement personnel unloaded the cargo, they would discover to their shock it was only 10,000. The frustration, he says, was made worse by the fact that he had no direct contact with AstraZeneca. 'To deal with such levels of unreliability and a complete lack of a client relationship. Just none. Here's what you're getting. Sorry, no, you're not getting that. It's next week. Actually it's not next week, it's the week after and it's half what you're expecting.' Constantly undercut by AstraZeneca, the HSE missed weekly target after weekly target. 'I hope that the word "game changer" is banned from the dictionary,' says Brian MacCraith.

MacCraith had to leave the despondency aside to focus on diplomacy. In conversations with the company's representatives, MacCraith pleaded for mercy. He told them on multiple occasions that the delays were prolonging Ireland's suffering. 'This is tens of thousands of people who are due to be vaccinated not getting their vaccine. This is not just about the impact of making a delivery change or a slight reduction in quantity. These are people at the end of it,' he'd say. He wanted AstraZeneca to know that they simply had to tell Ireland the bad news in advance if there were going to be supply problems. 'Don't leave us hanging on in the expectation,' he said. The message was heard but not heeded. Missed deliveries dogged the vaccine rollout for a long time to come.

The first three months of the year brought many dark days.

'This period has got the best and worst out of us,' says Paul Reid. 'The best of us – we got struck down again and took the hit and everybody just did what they had to do. But then the vaccination programme became this "it's me, it's my turn, not them, it's her, it's me, it's my daughter, it's not him over there". I'm just kind of going … Jesus.' He reflects on the demand in the early part of 2021: 'If we were doing this last June and July, I'd bet you we would have had a different issue in getting people to come forward for vaccinations. Whereas in February, March and April, we had everybody "I want it. Me! Me! Me!" you know?'

It was a long way from the excitement of late December when a small wooden pallet carting two cardboard boxes, no bigger than wine crates, was wheeled out of a Transit van and into CityWest. The Health Minister, Paul Reid and Brian MacCraith were there to greet it, snapping photos of this delivery that represented a way out of a year of sorrow and loss.

Looking at the tiny vials as they were stored in the HSE's newly commissioned giant fridges was an out-of-body moment of wonder. 'Is it not a strange fate that we should suffer so much fear and doubt for so small a thing?' in the words of Tolkien. In that first shipment were 9,750 doses, which came, as MacCraith remembers, when we 'were in serious, serious trouble' in the third wave. 'It was almost comic in terms of these little boxes and photographers chasing around flashing cameras at them but it meant that we were at the beginning of the journey.'

* * * *

On 19 February 2021, at Our Lady's Hospice in Harold's Cross, Dr Emer Holohan died. Tributes flowed in from across Irish public life. From the Government, from the Minister for Health, from Leo Varadkar, from old colleagues like Dr Marie Casey, who remembered Emer for 'her intelligence, her kindness and goodness ... and for her excellence in Public Health Medicine', and Dr Mai Mannix, who described her as a gifted doctor and a wonderful colleague.

On the day of Dr Holohan's death, her husband Tony had got into the family car with their two children, Clodagh and Ronan. The phone rang. It was Micheál Martin. He asked Holohan how the kids were. 'Well, they're actually here in the car with me at the moment, Taoiseach. They can both hear you.' Martin spoke to them both for ten minutes, sincerely expressing his sympathies.

Holohan returned to work on Monday, 20 April, getting through his first week, with another NPHET meeting on the horizon the following week as Ireland prepared its next steps in managing the pandemic response. On the Friday of his first week back, the Taoiseach called again. This wasn't Micheál Martin's usual check-in on the state of play and how his health advisers were feeling about moving on with reopening the country. It was a personal call. 'Welcome back, Tony,' he said, asking him how he was getting on and how things were at home. Martin sympathized with Holohan and asked him how Clodagh and Ronan were doing, mentioning them by name. Holohan, who had been through the wars with the Taoiseach over previous months, was blown away by the genuine sympathy and human solidarity shown by Martin, a man who has known what it's like to lose people you love.

'He put out a notice, you may not have seen it, in sympathy with Emer's passing and mentioned in it that she had done – which is true – that she had worked in the Department of Health as a public health trainee twenty years ago and worked on the health strategy. He mentioned that and I thought "Wow". It meant a lot.'

Holohan has received countless messages of support and sympathy from members of the public. He publicly expressed his gratitude in a note in the *Irish Times* ahead of what would have been Emer's birthday in May. He said his family had been 'humbled and greatly comforted by the extraordinary number of messages of condolence' received from so many people. 'What comes through so clearly in all the messages from those who knew Emer is her warmth, her kindness and her razor-sharp wit. Keep her in your hearts and prayers, remember her often and smile for the sunshine she brought.'

Like so many with terminal or serious illness, she lived in fear of Covid, says Holohan. Emer, Clodagh and Ronan spent a lot of precious time in their final months together.

Holohan, opening up, says his thoughts are complex about the situation. Funeral numbers and visitation were restricted. He was thankful, in a way, that they were able to go through it together, peacefully, without being overwhelmed. 'We did the funeral home on Saturday afternoon and we couldn't have anybody else other than immediate family and so we did it in blocks. So we did fifteen minutes, then my parents came, and then I have a couple of sisters, they each came separately, and then they all called to the door here, as they say. I was saying to the kids, when the three of us were up there with Emer when she was in the coffin and we were in the funeral home, I was saying: "If this was normal … if this wasn't … like there'd be just people coming in here and you'd be sitting there and you wouldn't have a chance." Whereas, we were able to spend fifteen minutes, it doesn't sound like a lot of time, but we were able to spend time and then leave when we were ready.'

Holohan's children, Emer's siblings, her father and Holohan's parents were the ten for the funeral mass. 'It felt very intimate and it felt very nice. That won't work for other people,' he says, 'because those numbers wouldn't work for other people but it actually gave us space and time that I don't think we would have had otherwise.'

In the weeks and months that have followed, Holohan has been blown away by the outpouring of support, the kindness of strangers, who have expressed their sympathy. The funeral home printed out a collection of the wishes left online through RIP.ie. The volume was extraordinary. Holohan has vowed to respond to every letter his family has received, cognisant of what everyone who wrote must have gone through too over the previous eighteen months.

There was a letter from a nun in a convent in the midlands, who was also suffering a long-term cancer and took inspiration from Emer's journey; there was a priest who started off with a beautifully written letter telling Holohan he had read the eulogy he gave at Emer's funeral. He quoted a passage from it and said he'd now incorporated it into his own funeral homilies. Turning over the page, the priest would go on to take issue with the wording of a Holohan press conference where he said 'the dogs on the street' in Donegal could see compliance was low. 'It was the best written letter of complaint I ever got,' says Holohan, appreciative of the time and the consideration.

Holohan says he's yet to make his way through all of the letters. 'I'm going to be responding to all of them at some point even if it takes me ten years,' he says.

* * * *

295

'Brian, I've some news for you.'

Brian MacCraith could tell by the tone in Paul Reid's voice that this wasn't going to be good news. By now, MacCraith's life was consumed entirely by the vaccine rollout. He'd come home late, and digest document after document, reading more and more information on the logistics, the vaccines and the evidence worldwide.

If anything had been learned over the initial months of managing vaccines it was that good news was fleeting and setbacks were all too regular. That morning's bolt from the blue – on Sunday, 14 March – which had kept Reid up throughout the night, was the decision by NIAC to pause the use of AstraZeneca following a report from Norway, which had identified four new cases of serious blood clotting in adults who had received the vaccine. By the time the news was officially confirmed, queues of healthcare workers at clinics across the country already knew.

Álainn Wong, a healthcare worker, was attending the vaccine clinic at Connolly Hospital in Blanchardstown. Thirty to forty healthcare workers, who had battled through the first, second and third waves of the virus, were greeted by the woman running the clinic, who informed them, 'I'm sorry, we've been told we can't administer the AstraZeneca vaccine from the Government. The clinic has been told to shut.' It was a demoralizing jolt for those queuing, people who had organized taxis, or long multi-leg public transport trips to get to the clinic.

Others, in the Cohort 4 category of people at very high risk from Covid-19 had their vaccinations cancelled too. For people who had cocooned and shielded for months, missing important family moments, isolating themselves from their society and their family, the whiplash of this decision nearly pushed many to the edge.

The Government and health service consistently hammered the line that 'supply is the only issue'. It wasn't.

Things started small with a minor controversy over 110 doses of vaccine being dumped at a nursing home in the East after being incorrectly stored, but public fury was soon centred on the stories of vaccinations out of sequence.

At the Coombe Women and Infants University Hospital in January, a consultant took doses from the hospital to vaccinate his family members at home. An independent review commissioned by the hospital into the vaccination of sixteen family members of staff found that doses were administered to one or more family members of eight staff.

In March, the *Irish Daily Mail*'s Craig Hughes uncovered the story that twenty teachers and staff at the elite fee-paying St Gerard's School in County Wicklow were given 'leftover' vaccines from the Beacon private hospital. Gerard's is the school that Beacon chief executive Michael Cullen's children attend. These stories, coming at a time of severe lockdown restrictions and with questions looming large about the vaccine rollout pace, lent themselves to a volatile situation which the Government failed to control.

Targets had been set. And the failure to meet them was a millstone around the coalition's neck. The Taoiseach, for example, confidently voiced a target of eighty per cent of the adult population to have had a first dose by the end of June, with around fifty-five per cent fully vaccinated. Privately, as Micheál Martin announced these figures, there was no small amount of shock in Health circles. They had seen this before in the testing debacle of the spring of 2020 – targets publicly being set for which they would be held accountable.

The issue of leaks from Cabinet had been churning around Government for a long time, but it was around March that the Greens at the Cabinet table found themselves aghast at how crucial decisions were being played out in the media before they had their chance to have their say. In late March, the Government took advice from NIAC and the CMO to change the rollout, once the over-65s were vaccinated, to an age-based allocation rather than one based on a mix of age and profession. The matter came to Cabinet almost without warning for some ministers.

'It was almost live tweeting at that stage. There was a long discussion that day and I feel what was leaked out to the news on Twitter that day influenced that discussion,' says one minister. 'I was furious after that meeting. It was a difficult issue and then you've this bullshit happening. I came in with a view and my view changed to some extent having heard the rationale put forward in Cabinet.' In several ministers' views, the decision taken that day was made too quickly, while it was later accepted wholesale, and the Cabinet was bounced into it as a result of it being reported as a *fait accompli* in the media. 'It wasn't fair to anyone – gardaí, teachers, the public – because it was a nuanced issue that required debate.'

Days later, the coalition almost came unstuck. AstraZeneca was paused for those under the age of sixty, while exports of Johnson & Johnson's single-dose Janssen vaccine, another 'game changer', were vetoed. The Government was staring down the barrel of missed deadlines. The buzzwords and hand-waving were not going to work any longer. A public tired of hearing how vaccines would 'ramp up' were on their knees.

Bogged down by the calamitous rollout of hotel-based quarantine for arrivals from a number of countries, struggling to manage expectations of the vaccine rollout, and with the longest lockdown yet lengthening day by day, the Cabinet met on Wednesday, 14 April to discuss the situation. The meeting was dour. There was a feeling of near-resignation among many ministers, some now convinced that the Government's race was run. The ministers who came together across the three rooms didn't speak before the meeting. It was funereal. 'It was over. I remember thinking fairly quickly about whether or not I'd be standing in the next election that day,' says one minister.

It was do or die for the Taoiseach. Micheál Martin was left in no doubt by his parliamentary party, by the opposition and by a growing sense of frustration from a beleaguered public. 'They were lining up for us,' Martin remembers. 'People are getting pissed off, they're fed up of lockdown, they hate us, open it up. All of that, you know.' Officials who were present when the Taoiseach met British Prime Minister Boris Johnson say he was envious when Johnson told him flippantly that he'd taken a 'punt' to prioritize wholly the first doses of vaccine. That strategy had paid off spectacularly for Britain in the first half of 2021, which only served to fan the flames of anger here. All the while, headlines in the London press goaded Europe for turning down the 'British vaccine'.

Ministers scribbled down figures, vainly clutching at some arrangement to see them out of this mess. The numbers didn't add up. The plan was crumbling around their heads. Micheál Martin put on a brave face, but there was a feeling of deep despondency drifting through the three rooms. The Taoiseach was called away to take an unexpected call from Brussels. When he returned he told his ministers, with barely concealed glee, that he had some very good news from Ursula von der Leyen, but he would hold off on telling them for fear that, once again, news would leak from the Cabinet table.

'Too late for that,' smirked Leo Varadkar, 'it's already online.' The EU had a new deal with Pfizer on production. Ireland was to receive a much-needed 540,000 doses.

Ministers who were present describe feelings of relief, euphoria, glee. There were suppressed yelps and fist pumps. One minister, a keen sports fan, compared it to conceding a last-minute goal in a Champions League final, only to see it scrapped by the Video Assistant Referee. They might get out of this yet.

The calculators and scraps of paper came out again as ministers figured out whether or not the June target was once again within reach. In any case, it's a moment now regarded across politics as a turning point in the malaise. But it would not be the last challenge.

As that week drew to a close, the Health Minister had reason to feel good. There was the Pfizer news; he had successfully negotiated the public health consultant contract, buying himself some much-needed brownie points with doctors across the country; and he had won his battle at Cabinet level with the Foreign Affairs Minister Simon Coveney over mandatory hotel quarantine. Things were looking up for the Greystones man. That was until he spoke to the *Irish Times*. In an interview with political editor Pat Leahy, Donnelly floated the suggestion that 18–30-year-olds might be bumped up the vaccine queue to stop the spread of the virus.

The reaction was thunderous. On the Saturday morning of publication, gardaí and teachers flooded their TDs' inboxes and loudly voiced their grievances. If they were being told to wait their turn for the sake of the science, this suggestion surely flew in the face of that. In messages across the senior vaccine rollout plan, members of the HSE and the Department of Health were astonished. 'What the *fuck*,' was the first reaction from one of the HSE managers, 'can't we go a single week without a gaffe?' It was an idea that was instantly rejected. Paul Reid had read about the suggestion in the papers on the way to the Helix where he was due to speak at the vaccine clinic. He was left with no choice but to publicly shoot it down, just as Acting Chief Medical Officer Dr Ronan Glynn had done in a meeting with Donnelly days before he conducted the interview with the *Irish Times*.

Members of the Fianna Fáil and Fine Gael parties railed against Donnelly. 'He was told on Friday that your man Glynn didn't think it was a good idea,' says one senior Fianna Fáil member. 'I got lots of emails about Stephen's plan. People don't normally contact their TDs on a Saturday. We said okay, we're going to do it on an age basis and then we're trying to tell teachers we're going to do the eighteen-year-old kids in your class first?'

That was as polite as the contributions got. Donnelly recanted the suggestion as just that – 'a suggestion'. One move he did make earlier on in the vaccine rollout did not get much coverage at the time but was, by many people's account, hugely important.

At the beginning of the plan, the initial move was shaping up to be a rollout starting in the nursing homes. That didn't happen. It changed on foot of advice that suggested hospital or clinical environments should be the first port of call. That continued into January, even as nursing homes sustained incalculable losses. 'We were going straight into nursing homes, they [NIAC] said no, you can't go into nursing homes, it has to be a clinical setting,' says Paul Reid. The advice had senior staff across Health and the HSE worried about the delay in getting to care facilities. It was the Health Minister who, on a solo run that wasn't warmly greeted by some in the sector at the time, urged Reid and the Task Force to get to work on the nursing homes immediately.

Some wonder whether, if the initial advice to protect the nursing homes first had been followed, more lives would have been saved. Others say there's no telling how much more desperate the hospital crisis might have become in the same time period if that had been the case. It's a moral dilemma on a huge scale. The responsibility of government and decision-making in such times boils down to such dilemmas.

As matters improved on vaccinations, the growing role of the Department of the Taoiseach in managing the pandemic was becoming more publicly apparent. In early April, Micheál Martin joined Paul Reid and Brian MacCraith on a tour of the vaccination centre at CityWest. They were announcing that almost one million people would have received a vaccine by the end of the day, and to give projections on the plan for Quarter 2. The Health Minister was not invited, and a hastily arranged photo opportunity at the Aviva Stadium was facilitated to give Donnelly face time with the media. The fact that Donnelly rarely shared a platform with the Taoiseach at Covid-related events any more was commented upon internally – although people close to the Health Minister say there were too many men in suits involved at most of these events anyway, with the trio of party leaders coming to the fore. Two HSE management team members say that Donnelly has sought to involve himself in announcements, looking for good news to put out there rather than having the HSE make the announcements themselves – which is a 'point of tension' between themselves and the Department. Rather than the HSE announcing the portal opening for new age brackets, it appeared in the Health Minister's Twitter feed.

As the months rolled on, Ireland ticked slowly through the age groups. Sixties, fifties, forties. Small protests, the largest of which, in July 2021, was about two thousand strong, were often organized by far-right political groups who threatened violence against politicians and medics. However, there was no sign of the anti-vaccine movements taking hold at the same level as in other Western countries.

One summer afternoon, a small group of demonstrators approached me outside the Department of Health, where I was removing my earpiece after a live broadcast on Virgin Media. Instinctively, as so many of us did whenever people came too close, I clutched for my face covering, throwing it on before they arrived beside me holding their banners and placards. 'Take that off you,' was the first thing they said. They were a group of five women, friends from different corners of the island. The youngest among them went straight for abuse. 'You're a fucking disgrace,' she spat, jabbing her finger at camera operator Eoin Kelly and me.

Passers-by glanced over, thinking better of stopping. We discussed their views, their concerns, and the wisdom of using abusive language against people they had never met in their lives. Some of the group were mothers, their own fears for their children exploited by misinformation online. Lies spread faster than the social networks could delete them; if, that is, they bothered to delete them at all. In the end, after what eventually became a respectful conversation, I wished them good health. I told them my own first vaccine appointment at my local GP's surgery was later that day. They warned me. 'I guarantee it, you'll be dead in two years if you put that in your body.'

Later, posting a selfie with my HSE vaccine card that evening, I scanned through the comments. '2 years Richard!!! Dont say we didnt warn you'. I paused and wondered. What happens to their small movement over those two years, when 2020 and 2021 are distant memories that so many of us will race to forget?

As the months wore on, a distant threat drew near. The Delta variant, first detected in India, threatened to undo the slow, steady progress of those dark months just as Ireland was finally getting its house in order. The HSE accelerated the vaccine rollout, pumping vials to centres and pharmacies like pistons on an engine. Take-up roared ahead of the European average. By 1 August, seventy-two per cent of the adult population had been fully vaccinated, creeping ahead of the United Kingdom's rate, which had dogged Ireland's vaccinators and HSE logistics teams all year. For them, it was sweet relief. Their efforts were paying off at last.

* * * *

In the Helix, joyful chatter filled the air. People in their seventies and eighties were meeting neighbours and old friends they hadn't seen since Leo Varadkar told them it was time to cocoon in March 2020. Now they were emerging from

303

the chrysalis of their own four walls, their lives once again taking wing in glorious technicolour of fluttering laughter and teary reunions.

Dr Maitiu Ó Faoláin told the med students at the reception desk to be at their warmest and friendliest. 'Have a smile on your faces, guys. You're the first social contact – you're a substitute for months of time they haven't been with grand-kids or anyone. Have a bit of fun checking them in ... but be quick about it, you're on the clock and you have forty seconds to do it.'

The GPs, looking after their own patients in the cubicles of the theatre floor, would ask their patients what it all meant to them. Eyes would tear up. One man said he was so excited to be able to visit his brother in Phibsboro. Even family members so close were kept so far apart in the year of Covid.

It was tiring work. Dr Maitiu Ó Faoláin would come home from nine hours coordinating, vaccinating and scurrying about in the Helix, sit on the sofa, his wife would hand him his reheated dinner and he'd keep working until two or three in the morning. 'For most of February, March and April I dreamt, slept, lived nothing but Covid – and nothing but the Helix.'

It was restorative for GPs like Ó Faoláin, who had spent the third wave in the eye of a storm, to be witness to a new hope. He thought back to Christmas Eve 2020, when people with telltale coughs decided not to get tested. His mind strayed back to New Year's Day, when he volunteered on call in the north-east, handling eighty calls over four hours and driving himself ninety kilometres each way, rubbing his eyes with tiredness behind the wheel.

'You weren't even looking to the end of the week back then, you were just looking to survive the day.' To go from that to being one of the 119 GPs personifying hope in the Helix was a glorious redemption.

Now, the upset calls of parents looking for tests for their

kids, or requests for urgent hospital transfers, had given way to the sound of families joking together as they spilled out onto the college campus, linking arms with their newly vaccinated parent or grandparent, a reminder of the connection that had been lost over the long months of lockdown. *Anois teacht an Earraigh, beidh an lá dúl chun shínead.* Spring had come at last.

Chapter 21: Moving On

St Mary's Hospital, Phoenix Park, Dublin, April 2021

The car thermometer reads 20 degrees and it feels every one of them. Another warm spring day. Just like it was last year when the sun beamed through the glaring glass at St Mary's. Things are very different from 2020, when staff faded under the weight of gowns and masks in the heat, in a crisis of such desperation. When families stood on the benches, their hands cupping their mouths, shouting their mother's name, desperate to be seen and heard; those same benches they now sit on with the loved one they're visiting. When residents, confused and frightened, couldn't see loved ones in their hour of need, now back to art classes and sitting out watching the deer munch the grass around the hospital grounds, pattering slowly around underneath the cherry blossoms.

Things didn't return to normal quickly. How could they? Twenty-four lives were lost to Covid in St Mary's in the spring of 2020; it is a scar that will never fade.

'It has affected them,' says healthcare assistant Alison Fitzgerald of the residents. 'Some of them were fearful to come out of their rooms.' Staff would ask residents to come down to the day room for a while. They were reluctant. But bit by bit, careful reassurance opened things up.

When St Mary's cleared its outbreak, a remembrance service

was held for those twenty-four lives that were lost. It was conducted virtually, a link sent to families of those who had died over those horrific months.

In previous years, branches on a remembrance tree would be dedicated to those who had died over the previous year. Last autumn, the staff at St Mary's planted two new trees, one near each of the buildings, to mark those they had lost and give staff and families a space to remember them. They're both apple trees, blooming into bright flower in April, a symbol of new life.

* * * *

A wild hydrangea now grows in West Cork in remembrance of Sheila Murphy. Another plant to symbolize a vibrant life.

For those who lost loved ones in the spring of 2020, when the pandemic first swept through the country, remembrance a year on was stifled by the same restrictions that were required to stem the tide and save more lives. It is a prolonged grief for those left behind. Conor Murphy, a year on from Sheila's passing, has taken to reliving old memories he has of his wife and life partner who changed his world and enriched so many others around Clonakilty.

In the late spring and early summer, Mary, his daughter, says, they started going on trips together to relive happy memories. They go for spins around the town, near the spot where Conor came crashing into Sheila's life so many years ago; out to Timoleague to see the old cottage where they lived in their first year of marriage. Conor remembers how Sheila, who was working at a home for boys with learning difficulties or who were orphaned, organized for three boys from the home to come up to the cottage with them for Christmas. It was their first Christmas as a married couple, and Sheila organized Santa for the kids. Memories like this have piled up on a Remembering Sheila Murphy Facebook group, followed by hundreds of people, each sharing their own story of a life well lived.

Remembrance is one thing. Accountability is another. Families like those of Rosie Hegarty and of Noreen Butler have called for a public inquiry into what happened in the nursing homes. Judith, Noreen's daughter, still spends nights overcome by the pain of her loss, staring at the ceiling at night, her mind racing with the upset. 'It's good to chat about it, sometimes I think it didn't happen at all. It's about protecting ourselves because if you thought about it too much, it can be very overwhelming.'

Until that point, when an inquiry delivers its final say, moving on will be difficult.

Driving through a village on her way to Cork, Dr Mary Favier checked her mirrors. Something caught her eye. It was a faded poster, battered and worn by months in the wind and rain. 'Support our healthcare heroes'. 'I just thought, well, that is so last year,' she says.

It's a point that was driven home directly to politicians at the Oireachtas Health Committee in February 2021 by Dr Gabrielle Colleran, a consultant radiologist at the National Maternity Hospital. While politicians clapped for frontline workers, little had been done to lessen their burden. She told the committee that there was no plan for healthcare workers' children. 'I got home at nine-fifteen p.m. on Monday last night, and my seven-year-old was sitting there with her *Abair Liom* on the table, waiting to do her Irish homework with me. I burst into tears. I had nothing left to give. She is stressed because she is falling behind. The anxiety is through the roof. We are not working from home, we are not there to support our children. We feel we have been abandoned by the State at exactly the time when we have all stepped up.' Her message hit home with thousands of families of healthcare workers across the country.

The ones who risked their lives, who saw their colleagues and friends get sick and not return for weeks or months with long Covid. The frontline heroes were left to pick up the pieces on the home front too.

Everyone involved in Government knows there will be an inquiry. Publicly they support and champion it. But there are grumblings that it will turn into a 'witch hunt'. Micheál Martin believes it's important that it doesn't become an interrogation. 'Officials who are at the helm need to know this isn't a blame game for the next time because they'll get more cautious and operate on a "protect my backside" approach in a subsequent crisis.'

Many involved in the Department of Health's response are wary about the atmosphere at such inquiries, wondering if they will go the same way as the Oireachtas Covid Committee meetings of 2020. Some civil servants look at those meetings and see a lot of grandstanding, TDs looking for their moment in the spotlight, shouting and roaring, giving themselves plenty of fodder for their social media channels. They watched those meetings, attended by Tony Holohan and Ronan Glynn and others, and believe it did 'untold damage in terms of the overall response'. One senior Health civil servant says that while many deputies asked valid questions, the atmosphere of attack and defence on committees will not lead to accountability or to any real learning. 'If we keep going the way we're going, no one will ever be willing to take a risk. We won't improve, we won't innovate change.'

At a HSE briefing on Thursday, 13 May, a chipper Paul Reid made reference to the lightened national mood as the country opened up and the vaccine programme ground through the gears. He felt so confident in the situation that he started using football metaphors, describing Ireland as being 2–0 up against Covid, with the vaccines 'knocking in the goals'.

The very next day the news of the largest cyber attack in the history of the State broke. Russian-based hackers had conducted

309

a ransomware operation against the HSE. Imaging, diagnostics, labs, emails and more were all lost. Just as things were beginning to improve, the heavy burden of fifteen months of pandemic care slowly easing across an exhausted health service, nurses and doctors were thrown back immediately to the 1970s. The disruption in many units was worse than Covid itself.

For public health teams it was one of the most difficult times of the pandemic. In Galway, Dr Breda Smyth and her team were scrambling between WhatsApp groups, pulling together notes, scribbling data in copybooks. 'If someone was working on a case and they had a day off, then it was dependent on someone else remembering that person was dealing with that specific case. It was a nightmare, an absolute nightmare.' The cyber attack exposed the dependence in the health service on outdated systems. Facilities like the Children's Health Ireland hospitals relied on a number of computers that dated back to the 1990s. Going back through the pandemic, the crash of the close contact tracing network in October 2020 and the reliance on the CIDR system for case reporting highlighted an IT system that was not 'match fit', in the words of Paul Reid, for what it would need to do over the course of the pandemic.

The HPSC, Ireland's agency responsible for monitoring the spread of communicable diseases, went into the pandemic relying on this software and it suffered the same crisis in retention and recruitment as the public health departments.

Dr Niall Conroy, a Dubliner who is a consultant in public health medicine, left Ireland for Australia in early 2020 before the onset of the pandemic. Looking at the Irish response through the prism of a well-funded public health system has infuriated him at times. 'In Australia, there would be a lot of work going into pandemic planning. That didn't happen in Ireland. One of the reasons was because they couldn't recruit somebody to the directorship for the HPSC. There were people acting in the role and that's their role. If you wanted to pick Ireland's pandemic planner, our Tony Fauci, it's the director of the HPSC and when people are in there transiently or they're not particularly empowered to do their job, then [pandemic planning is] never going to happen,' he says. 'There are very good people who are very, very capable of planning for a pandemic in Ireland. We just didn't have enough of them. Ireland has the expertise to do it. And I suspect after this we'll see a more Australia-style annual stress-testing of the response.'

While hopes rose as summer came, the warm sun brought diners to city streets in Dublin, Galway and, particularly, Cork, which had pedestrianized seventeen streets and lanes for outdoor dining. It brought a touch of a continental al fresco atmosphere to Ireland's streetscapes and breathed new vibrancy and oxygen in as traffic took a detour out.

There was a feeling as June came that all of this was finally going to plan. The cities were no longer in the sole possession of urban foxes and lonely Garda patrols. It certainly made Finance Minister Paschal Donohoe's walks around the capital all the more cheerful than they had been. A noted bookworm, frequently publishing reviews in the *Irish Times*, Donohoe would often ask journalists what they'd been reading and throw in a few suggestions for them. One book he regularly pushed on me, at the end of press conferences or in chance meetings around Merrion Street, was Albert Camus' *The Plague*, which he had sought out in the early days of the emergency. It's been a near-constant on his desk ever since, often dipped into in the dark hours when the rolling tide of the pandemic came back in and the Government's plans were dashed. 'Indeed it could be said that once the faintest stirring of hope became possible, the dominion of the plague was ended.'

The summer brought with it a hope that Ireland was through the worst of a virus that would simply not go away, eyes turning to the next challenges and moving on. Moving on, however, is never simple. Left behind in the dust of a health service that reconfigured itself completely to wrestle with coronavirus were countless long-term problems, while new ones quietly surfaced.

As troops were diverted to man the battlements against Covid, waiting lists grew behind the walls. Cancer. Maternity care. Scans.

GPs noted a rise in mental health issues presenting amongst their patients, particularly young adults. Dr Amy Morgan, in her Drogheda practice, watched the problem grow and grow. 'It almost felt on any given day, it was seventy, maybe eighty per cent of what you were seeing, particularly in young people.' She worried. People were presenting for the first time with eating disorders. Students who had left school for college in Dublin or further afield were back living at home with their parents for the first time in a long time. 'They wouldn't have been at home for such a protracted period of time,' Dr Morgan says. 'They were coming in with a family member, you know, who is now able to see this first-hand.'

It was upsetting. Amy was handling these calls from families she had known for years and the pain that was bubbling up underneath was affecting so many of them. She thought about how much of their lives had been uprooted. Teenagers missing the last days of their secondary school lives – no graduations, no debs, no Leaving Cert holidays. Those in college had missed out on freshers' weeks, new experiences and meeting new people and connections that could last a lifetime, in a new environment where they could develop and grow on their own. 'It was really tough. Seeing people and seeing their family members who didn't know this was going on. These were kids who had never presented before. Maybe it was there all along and the pandemic exposed that. It was really a sense of hopelessness.'

She couldn't tell what was ahead for those young people after they had left her office – she had to move on immediately to the next patient. But as she sat and gave herself the time to think when she got home and fell into the sofa, she couldn't help but worry about the lack of supports that were available pre-pandemic, and how her patients would cope after the virus had gone.

Key members of the HSE's management team talk with sincere regrets about the 'things to have been missed' during the pandemic. Professor Martin Cormican, the HSE's national lead on infection control, is pensive as he looks back on the first eighteen months of the pandemic in Ireland. 'The one thing that stands out in my mind is the harm we've done to people that we didn't mean to do,' he says. 'I don't mean any one person now but I think that some people with good intentions probably took infection prevention and control in a way that I would have never thought about it. Meaning well did great and unnecessary harm by taking things too far.'

I ask if this is a reference to end-of-life visits? To partners who have been locked out of crucial appointments with their loved one and child in maternity hospitals? 'A number of things,' he says. 'A number of things. You know more than I that things were brought to our attention where we said, "We never said that. We never wanted our guidance to be interpreted in that way. That's not what we meant."' He is commiserative about this. He makes sure that I do not interpret his words to mean that anyone was doing it out of malice. 'The people who have made these mistakes, it's not that they were bad people. They were frightened. They were often trying to do the right thing. But you know, I think that we, as a society and as a healthcare system both, I think we could have been kinder to each other.'

'Do you know *Moby Dick*?' says a senior NPHET member. 'There were elements of the Captain Ahab about it. The captain of the ship lost sight; all he saw was the whale. There was enormous secondary harm, without doubt. Ultimately, the cause was the virus but there was secondary harm that will be with us for years to come. There was illness, cancer presentations ... I blame myself here too but they never displayed encouragement, there was never a culture of looking at the secondary harm sufficiently. It's the single biggest thing. Where was the subgroup? Where was the entity looking at the harm ensuing from chasing the whale?'

The Irish Cancer Society estimates that some 2,000 invasive cancers may have been missed throughout 2020 as a result of the pandemic. People refused to go to their GP; during the first lockdown one in four people with health concerns did not attend their local doctor. Preparations, the Society says, must be made now for a cancer epidemic in the coming years.

Covid too comes with its own health burden. Thousands of people are suffering long-term impacts. What has become known as long Covid affects as many as one in seven people infected with the virus, with impacts lasting twelve weeks or longer.

Some impacts are small-scale, however unpleasant, like the experience of UCD student Lauren Maunsell, who for months after her infection cried after eating meals – an ongoing change to her sense of taste and smell makes almost everything taste like 'rotting meat'. Others, suffering from 'brain fog' months after their illness, have stopped driving for fear of forgetting how to get home or being involved in a crash. Another woman, interviewed for Virgin Media News, remembers going to the bathroom one night and forgetting how to work the light switch. Other long-term impacts are even more debilitating.

Ciaran O'Neill, a hotel manager living in Meath, was admitted to Tallaght Hospital with Covid in March 2020, brought in by his partner Bella unable to speak, his sister crying down the phone on loudspeaker to him as they arrived at the emergency department. The next day he was told by a doctor that he would be put to sleep and ventilated to help his lungs. He texted his family, including his fourteen-year-old son, to tell them goodbye, that he might never see them again. He was in an induced coma for sixteen days. He has never fully recovered.

The battle only really began when he returned home to Enfield. His breathing suffered. Heart palpitations kept him awake until the small hours of the morning, wondering if he was going to die. What stuck around the longest has been the nerve damage. His medics aren't sure if it resulted from proning in ICU or from losing two stone in his time in hospital. It changed his life by making him a prisoner to his own recovery. He struggled to climb flights of stairs. In excruciating pain, he sobbed as he dragged his leg behind him. He couldn't hold a cup of tea without scalding himself. He was on multiple painkillers every single day. It was overwhelming. Ciaran suffered PTSD, his mind racing back to the nightmares and delirium he experienced when he was on the ventilator. He couldn't help scrolling back through the texts he sent in 2020, in what he felt were his dying moments, to his partner, his son, his family. It's far too much to process. His psychologist at Tallaght Hospital recommended he try to get back to work before the first anniversary of his admission. It wasn't to be. Everything in March 2021 was coloured by the fact that 'this day last year' he was in a coma, struggling to keep breath in his body.

'Will I ever get back?' is a question he's asked himself so many times. It's one that people who regularly visit the Covid Cases Ireland page on Facebook ask themselves and peers, all going through terrifying symptoms, looking for people who have been through it and can relate to the loneliness and sorrow associated with what the virus left behind in their bodies. The pandemic continues to leave so many in its wake, officially 'recovered' but still not getting better.

Dr Tony Holohan knows that for many people the virus will never end. 'There's a burden for people who have lost people, for people who have lost jobs or businesses. These are things you can't easily recover from or forget,' he says. His spats with the HSE on the role of public health departments, regional response teams with autonomy to take meaningful actions in the event of outbreaks, are close to the top of his mind. While politicians and civil servants say the lessons will be learnt from Covid, there is a lingering fear that when it's gone, it'll be forgotten. Will antiquated IT systems be replaced many years after an overhaul was first mooted? Will Ireland bring itself up to international standards in pandemic response planning? Will our hospitals, struggling for headroom in wards and ICUs in a non-pandemic situation ever see the radical change to bring much-needed capacity to the frontlines? These are all questions that will remain for some time.

Whitty Building, the Mater Hospital

The doctor stands in the lift, the doors closing in front of her face. Her department, Gastroenterology, is on Level 4. She closes her eyes sometimes when she's carried up to the fourth floor, hoping the lift won't stop at ICU on Level 3. Every day for the first few months the lift trips were the hardest when the PA system's voice announced 'Level 3'. Dr Sammar Ali remembers everything about the lifts all too well: the panicked journeys with her family to visit her father as he lay on a ventilator, walking past the same security guards and staff as they did on those dreadful summer days, following the same footpaths, the same stairs.

On her very first day of work last January, in the middle of the third wave, she was confronted with so many memories. The doors opened on Level 3 and she looked out to the ICU waiting room, seeing the patterned fabric of the same gown her father had worn. Her heart dropped to the ground.

A deep breath. Close your eyes. Carry on. This was everything her father had prepared her for. She wished he was here now to see her and guide her.

Sammar's first days were the hardest. She'd always imagined that they'd be spent working alongside her father, just as they had planned. Most of her colleagues had started at the change-over in July. They were able to call up whatever they needed on the computer in an instant. She had to ask. Sammar felt awkward, a little out of place in a hospital that was operating at its usual breakneck pace and faster. The lift trips continued. 'Just one more floor, just one more floor,' Sammar would tell herself. Whenever they had a patient who needed to go to ICU, she would feel a longing to go to the room in which her father had spent his final weeks. Praying for some miracle that he would still be there, smiling and waiting for her to arrive.

While almost all of the doctors in the Mater know about Dr Syed Waqqar Ali, fewer knew this was his daughter working among them. One day the call of her father's room pulled her in. She went right up to the door and looked in, letting the memories wash over her. 'Are you okay, Sammar?' asked one of the ICU staff.

'What? Yes, no, I'm okay.'

'No, are you okay, Sammar?'

Sammar wasn't paying much attention – this person obviously knew her from somewhere. It was a medic who had cared for her dad. 'I understand how hard this must be,' she said. 'I understand why you're standing where you're standing right now.' She rubbed Sammar's shoulder. Sammar bit her lip and felt her eyes well up behind her goggles.

Like all doctors, Sammar has lost patients too. The first was the hardest. She stood outside the room just like her family had done in July, waiting to be cleared to enter. So much was the same. The silence. The sombre atmosphere. The window of the hospital room even faced the same way as her dad's. Sammar's heart started to race again, and climb steadily into her mouth. She had to step out.

The emotional response has been hard. It has been intense. But it reminds Sammar why she's here, the journey she has started out on. People have shown kindness too. Some people sent cards when they learned she was working at the Mater. In March, she sat on her break opening some of the envelopes that had gathered. Inside one was a printout. It was her Irish Medical Council registration page right alongside her father's. It's a gesture she'll never forget and one that touched her heart, lifting it to a new place of courage.

Sammar goes through the same doors every day. Often working in the same emergency department her father worked in, alongside the same nurses, doctors, HCAs he worked alongside. She togs out in her PPE and has come to a place where she feels pride. She is proud she pulled herself to where she wanted to be. Every day she feels her father behind her. Still offering encouragement and wisdom. Still waiting to hear about her day.

'Every time I've gone up that lift, I've been a little bit braver.' The lift doors open. Level 4. Time to go to work. Just as she said last spring, when she stood outside her home with her siblings to remember the father who had given them so much and had inspired so many.

'There is still a Dr Ali in the Mater and she will carry on his legacy.'

* * * *

It was the last day of July, teenagers shuffled along together outside CityWest, accompanied by their mams taking embarrassing videos for posterity. 'You'll want to remember this in years to come.'

318

It was the first day of walk-in vaccinations at thirty-eight centres across Ireland. Hundreds and hundreds of people, aged from sixteen up, queued from 6 a.m. for their first doses, their ticket for the climb out of this long national nightmare. The scene was replicated in Croke Park and Carndonagh, Castleblayney and Kilkenny, in Clonmel and Clonguish. More than ten thousand vaccinations were carried out that day, predominantly on younger people who gave up so much of their lives so that others might live.

Inside the hall at CityWest, as the line snaked around him, student Nelson Aguilar, from Bolivia, pulled up his seat at the piano, adjusted his mask and played. The chatter in the hall faded out as he lost himself in a tune that had come to mean so much to him. It was his own arrangement of 'Sometimes You Can't Make it on Your Own', written by U2's Bono about the passing of his father in 2001. Sitting atop the piano was his iPad propped up on its stand with a photo of Nelson sharing a bench with his dad Cesar back home. Cesar died from Covid in 2020. This was his tribute to his father, and to his young peers doing their bit to keep more parents from passing away.

At the peak of Covid, 605,839 people were in receipt of Pandemic Unemployment Payments. By 1 August, 5,849,924 vaccines had been administered in the Republic, 302,074 cases had been confirmed and 5,035 lives had been lost to the coronavirus.

At the time of writing, Ireland is still not out of the woods and the threat of new variants remains. The true cost of the virus will not be known for many years. In truth, it may never truly be known. How can you calculate what might have been but never was? There were so many memories that were yet to be made. All the happy anniversaries. All the babies born with both their beaming parents present. All the first dances. All the goodbyes in their own time. They are all lost to a phantom.

In communities ravaged by the virus, the healing is only just beginning. To walk down the main street in your nearest town is to be met with familiar and unfamiliar faces and not know what any of us have been through, what personal toll the virus took on us. The wounds of the long winter will take many years to heal. No memorials are yet built, no major commemorations have taken place. The tragedy that happened will come to the fore. Ireland must begin to remember.

Leabharlanna Poiblí Chathair Baile Átha Cliath
Dublin City Public Libraries

Acknowledgements

Without the honesty and openness of dozens of healthcare workers across the country, this book wouldn't exist. Thank you to each and every person who gave up so much time and allowed me into their experiences of a pandemic year. I am eternally grateful.

Thank you to Conor Nagle at HarperCollins Ireland, who first approached me to try my hand at writing back in January 2021. I could never have possibly imagined the volume of work and the ups and downs that would follow on the long road to print. His reassurance, support and belief in the value of this project has been steadfast and has steered me through moments when I thought we'd never make it across the line.

To Catherine Gough, Jane Rogers and Kerri Ward, whose expert advice turned streams of consciousness into a finished manuscript and who were ever patient and kind with their time and their thoughtful wisdom.

A heartfelt thanks to Patricia McVeigh for guiding me through the maelstrom between announcement and launch and whose unwavering positivity was a wonderful boost throughout the process.

Leah Foley of the Transcription Shop, I can't begin to thank you enough for the time you committed to this book, the scores of interviews you turned around so quickly and for being one of the few humans I could talk to about the project for so long. You are a star and I hope we work together again.

To Mick McCaffrey, my Head of News and Sport, for backing me from the beginning and for giving the book his seal of approval. To everyone in Virgin Media News, including editors Joe Walsh and Brian Daly; but particularly Zara King and Gavan Reilly. Our friendship, our WhatsApps and our chats carried us through the dark times of the pandemic. Their fact checks and feedback was crucial to getting the job done.

Thank you to Lisa Coen for contractual advice.

To my mother, Liz, and my brother Jeffrey, for their love and encouragement and for their understanding about the demands on time with writing and editing. I hope to make up for lost time and missed visits very soon.

Most of all, I'd like to thank Louise O'Neill. From the very beginning, you have given me so much inspiration, emotional support, guidance and love. A virus separated us for so much of the last two years, but your advice helped me to find my voice and kept me going on the long nights of writing and editing. This wouldn't have come close to happening without you. Thank you.